Handbook of General Surgical Emergencies

Sam Mehta
Specialist Registrar
General Surgery, Wessex Deanery

Andrew Hindmarsh
Specialist Registrar
General Surgery, Eastern Deanery

and

Leila Rees
Senior House Officer
General Surgery, Norfolk and Norwich University Hospital

Radcliffe Publishing
Oxford • Seattle

Radcliffe Publishing Ltd
18 Marcham Road
Abingdon
Oxon OX14 1AA
United Kingdom

www.radcliffe-oxford.com
Electronic catalogue and worldwide online ordering facility.

British Library Cataloguing in Publication Data

A catalogue record for this book is available from the British Library.

ISBN-10 1 85775 746 7
ISBN-13 978 1 85775 746 0

Typeset by Advance Typesetting Ltd, Oxford
Printed and bound by TJ International Ltd, Padstow, Cornwall

Contents

Preface

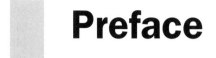

This book is intended as a pocket-sized resource for medical students and professionals working either in the accident and emergency department or in surgical admissions units.

We decided to write it because we felt that the handbooks currently available do not comprehensively cover the management of the acute surgical patient. Our handbook has been designed to provide an easy and quick portal of information for clinicians. It will also be useful as a revision aid for surgical examinations. Most topics are covered over two to four pages and should provide what you need to know to diagnose and treat patients when they first come into hospital.

The chapters do not cover each condition exhaustively and are not intended as a substitute for clinical judgement. Rather, we have tried to include as much relevant information as possible. For each topic we have performed a thorough literature review and incorporated evidence to support management strategies outlined in each chapter.

Sam Mehta
Andrew Hindmarsh
Leila Rees
January 2006

Glossary

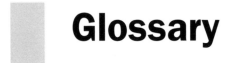

AAA	Abdominal aortic aneurysm
ABC	Airway breathing circulation
ABG	Arterial blood gas
ABPI	Ankle brachial pressure index
ADH	Anti-diuretic hormone
A&E	Accident and emergency
AF	Atrial fibrillation
AIDS	Acquired immune deficiency syndrome
ALP	Alkaline phosphatase
ALS	Advanced life support
ALT	Alanine aminotransferase
A–P	Anterior–posterior
APACHE	Acute Physiology and Chronic Health Evaluation
APTT	Activated partial thromboplastin time
ARDS	Adult respiratory distress syndrome
ASA	American Society of Anesthesiologists
AST	Asparate aminotransferase
ATLS	Advanced trauma life support
AXR	Abdominal X-ray
β-HCG	β-human chorionic gonadotrophin
BLS	Basic life support
BP	Blood pressure
BPH	Benign prostatic hypertrophy
CBD	Common bile duct
CNS	Central nervous system
COPD	Chronic obstructive pulmonary disease
CPAP	Continuous positive airway pressure
CRP	C-reactive protein
CPR	Cardiopulmonary resuscitation
CSF	Cerebrospinal fluid
CT	Computerised tomography
CVA	Cerebrovascular accident
CVP	Central venous pressure
CXR	Chest X-ray
DA	Dopamine
DIC	Disseminated intravascular coagulation
DM	Diabetes mellitus

DoH	Department of Health
2,3-DPG	2,3-diphosphoglycerate
DRE	Digital rectal examination
DU	Duodenal ulcer
DVT	Deep venous thrombosis
EBS	Evidence-based surgery
ECG	Electrocardiogram
ECHO	Echocardiogram
ENT	Ear, nose and throat
EOSIN	Eosinophils
ERCP	Endoscopic retrograde cholangiopancreatography
ESR	Erythrocyte sedimentation rate
ESWL	Extracorporeal shock wave lithotripsy
EUA	Examination under anaesthesia
FBC	Full blood count
FFP	Fresh frozen plasma
FNA	Fine needle aspiration
G&S	Group and save
GA	General anaesthesia/anaesthetic
GCS	Glasgow Coma Scale
GI	Gastrointestinal
GP	General practitioner
γ-GT	γ-glutamyl transferase
GU	Gastric ulcer
HAS	Human albumin solution
Hb	Haemoglobin
HCG	Human chorionic gonadotrophin
Hct	Haematocrit
HDU	High-dependency unit
HIV	Human immunodeficiency virus
IBD	Inflammatory bowel disease
ICAM	Intercellular adhesion molecule
ICP	Intracranial pressure
IDDM	Insulin-dependent diabetes mellitus
IgE	Immunoglobulin E
IL	Interleukin
INR	International normalised ratio
ITU	Intensive therapy unit
IUCD	Intra-uterine contraceptive device
i.v.	Intravenous
IVC	Inferior vena cava
IVU	Intravenous urogram
JVP	Jugular venous pressure
KUB	Kidney ureter bladder (X-ray)

LA	Local anaesthesia/anaesthetic
LDH	Lactate dehydrogenase
LFTs	Liver function tests
LIF	Left iliac fossa
LMWH	Low-molecular-weight heparin
LOC	Loss of consciousness
LUQ	Left upper quadrant
LUTS	Lower urinary tract symptoms
LYMPH	Lymphocytes
MC&S	Microscopy culture and sensitivity
MCV	Mean cell volume
MI	Myocardial infarction
MODS	Multi-organ dysfunction syndrome
MOF	Multi-organ failure
MRA	Magnetic resonance angiography
MRCP	Magnetic resonance cholangiopancreatography
MRI	Magnetic resonance imaging
MRSA	Methicillin-resistant *Staphylococcus aureus*
MST	Morphine sulphate tablets
MSU	Mid-stream urine
NBM	Nil by mouth
NCEPOD	National Confidential Enquiry into Peri-Operative Deaths
NEUT	Neutrophils
NG tube	Naso-gastric tube
NICE	National Institute for Clinical Excellence
NIDDM	Non-insulin-dependent diabetes mellitus
NIPPV	Non-invasive positive pressure ventilation
NSAID	Non-steroidal anti-inflammatory drug
OCP	Oral contraceptive pill
OGD	Oesophago-gastro-duodenoscopy
PA	Pulmonary artery
PAD	Phlegmasia alba dolens
PCA	Patient-controlled analgesia
PCD	Phlegmasia cerulea dolens
PCNL	Percutaneous nephrolithotomy
PE	Pulmonary embolus/embolism
PEEP	Positive end-expiratory pressure
PEG	Percutaneous endoscopic gastrostomy
PICC	Peripherally inserted central catheter
PID	Pelvic inflammatory disease
PLTS	Platelets
PPI	Proton pump inhibitor
PR	*Per rectum*
PSA	Prostate-specific antigen

PT	Prothrombin time
PUJ	Pelviureteric junction
RIF	Right iliac fossa
RR	Respiratory rate
RTA	Road traffic accident
RUQ	Right upper quadrant
SEPS	Sub-fascial endoscopic perforator surgery
SIRS	Systemic inflammatory response syndrome
SMA	Superior mesenteric artery
SOB	Shortness of breath
SSI	Surgical site infection
SVR	Systemic vascular resistance
TB	Tuberculosis
TCC	Transitional cell carcinoma
TED	Thromboembolic deterrent
TIPSS	Transjugular intrahepatic porto-systemic shunt
TNF	Tumour necrosis factor
TOE	Trans-oesophageal echocardiogram
TPN	Total parenteral nutrition
TRALI	Transfusion-related acute lung injury
TT	Thrombin time
U&Es	Urea and electrolytes
UC	Ulcerative colitis
URTI	Upper respiratory tract infection
USS	Ultrasound scan
UTI	Urinary tract infection
VF	Ventricular failure
VT	Ventricular tachycardia
V/Q	Ventilation/perfusion (scan)
vWF	von Willebrand factor
WBC	White blood cell count

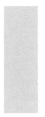

Chapter 1
Surviving 'on take'

Surviving 'on take'

Different hospitals adopt different policies with regard to who carries the on-call bleep, from the consultant to the most junior member of the team. Remember to be courteous and helpful to all general practitioners (GPs) who refer patients. Being rude on the phone not only wastes time and energy but may lead to negative feedback being relayed to your consultant.

GP admissions should be seen as soon as they arrive. This is important because you may receive a patient later who is critically unwell, and requires a great deal of time and investment. Keep a list that includes details of the expected patients, provisional diagnoses, any outstanding investigations and management plans. This will be particularly useful at handover times.

Working with the nursing staff

A positive relationship between surgeons and nurses is vital when looking after patients. Nurses can make your life much easier, so co-operate with them.

The respective roles of doctors and nurses have changed substantially in the last few years. Some nurses are now more specialised in certain areas, and increasingly take on some traditional 'doctor' roles.

Remember that nurses may have far more experience in dealing with patients from a practical viewpoint than you do. Therefore if you aren't sure ask for their help. In addition remember that many of the nurses may know about particular consultants' traits and behaviours.

Always communicate and liaise with whoever is looking after the patient, so that they have a clear idea of the diagnosis and plan of action. Many patients may feel more comfortable discussing their anxieties and questions with the nursing staff rather than clinicians.

One of the critical points of concern in the doctor/nurse relationship is time. Remember that everyone is under pressure. The nurse in question may be too busy to carry out everything you ask. Try and help out as much as possible. When you are similarly busy these same nurses will help you.

Working with the casualty department

It is important to establish a good relationship with the casualty department: they will be the source of many of your referrals and if you are polite and attend promptly they will be more likely to help you in return.

Remember:

- accident and emergency (A&E) staff are often busier than you and have different priorities. Their aim is to diagnose, stabilise and refer appropriately, and so they may not have requested all the specialist investigations you require
- when taking a referral establish who you are speaking to. The A&E doctor may not have as much experience in dealing with general surgical problems as you. However, never assume you know more than them
- if you are in doubt about the appropriateness of a referral try speaking to senior A&E staff. They will be able to tell you which specialties are available to deal with patients who have a particular diagnosis at your hospital. It is often quicker and easier for you to go and see the patient yourself if the diagnosis is unclear
- A&E departments often have protocols to follow – find out what they are
- waiting time restrictions are imposed on the A&E department and can be frustrating for them as well as you. Consequently, you may have to be flexible with regard to where you see the patient, and this can result in having to admit patients for a short period of time to complete your assessment.

Working with the radiology department

Plain radiographs should be organised as and when necessary. Abdominal X-rays are still over-ordered and generally have a low diagnostic yield. Indiscriminate ordering of X-rays wastes time and may be harmful to the patient.[1] It must be clear on the request card why you are ordering an X-ray. More importantly somebody should look at the film(s) as soon as they arrive back on the ward. A recent study has shown that most chest X-rays on acute *medical* admissions are not looked at until the following post-take ward round.[2] This is unacceptable in surgery.

Radiological workload has increased substantially over the last few years with advancing technology. There are more computerised tomography (CT) and magnetic resonance imaging (MRI) requests, and the field of interventional radiology is expanding. The on-call radiologist will be very busy, so ensure that

---

1   IRMER regulations (2000) www.doh.gov.uk (accessed 1 November 2005). Both the clinician ordering a radiological test and the radiographer ordering it can be held responsible for unnecessary radiation exposure to the patient. For this reason radiographers may question your request if the indication is not clear.
2   Nayak S and Lindsay KA (2004) Evaluation of the use of the X-ray department with regard to plain chest radiography on acute general medical admissions in the context of recently introduced UK guidelines. *Emerg Radiol* 10: 314–17.

all specialist investigations are justified, and discuss with your seniors before requesting them. If possible go and discuss the reasons for the request face-to-face rather than by telephone. They may be able to answer the same clinical question using a quicker, simpler or more accurate test.

The following information should be imparted to the radiologist:

- patient details with the appropriate form filled in
- why the patient needs the imaging, and in particular how the results may alter management. Give as much clinical information as possible
- who sanctioned the request
- how urgent the request is (i.e. immediately or later that day).

Radiologists may say 'no' if they are not convinced that the investigation is required or that it will alter management. In this case talk to your immediate senior and let him/her take things further.

Types of investigations

The following three investigations are commonly requested in acute general surgery.

Ultrasound

Ultrasound is useful in evaluating and diagnosing hepatobiliary, pancreatic, vascular and gynaecological pathology. It is an operator-dependent investigation. There is evidence that abdominal ultrasound may be a useful tool in the hands of surgeons with appropriate training. However this practice has not become commonplace in the UK.

Computerised tomography (CT)

Early abdominal CT in patients presenting with an acute abdomen has been shown to reduce hospital stay and perhaps mortality.[3] Disadvantages of CT include lack of resources and radiation dosage. When ordering a CT, ensure that the radiologist understands what you are looking for, since the type of scan is tailored to provide the best sensitivity and specificity. This may involve oral or intravenous (i.v.) contrast.

---

3   Ng CS, Watson CJ, Palmer CR *et al.* (2002) Evaluation of early abdominopelvic computed tomography in patients with acute abdominal pain of unknown cause: prospective randomised study. *BMJ* **325**: 1387.

Contrast examinations

- *Enteral contrast* may be given orally for a swallow or follow-through, or rectally. It may be barium or gastrograffin. Gastrograffin is used in the acute setting because it is water soluble and does not preclude subsequent surgery
- *Intravenous contrast* may be used for CT scanning, intravenous urogram (IVU) and angiography. Mention any allergies or renal impairment on the request form. Asthmatics may need steroid cover. Metformin should be stopped at least 48 h beforehand.

Working with anaesthetists

The surgeon and anaesthetist comprise the core medical team responsible for the management of the acute surgical patient. As well as giving the anaesthetic to facilitate surgery, the anaesthetist has a valuable role in both the pre- and post-operative management of the unstable patient and in pain control. It is therefore important to involve the anaesthetist at an early stage.

When contacting the anaesthetist about a patient they will expect you to tell them:

- the current problem
- how unwell the patient is
- the urgency of surgery
- your management so far
- a full medical history including current medications
- results of baseline investigations, e.g. full blood count (FBC), urea and electrolytes (U&Es), Clotting and arterial blood gases (ABGs).

You must also ensure additional investigations such as electrocardiogram (ECG) and chest X-ray (CXR) (if appropriate) have been performed and are available.

A conflict that frequently occurs between the surgeon and anaesthetist is the timing of surgery for patients with urgent but non-life-threatening conditions who present at night. Many of these patients are elderly with co-existing disease and are therefore at higher risk of developing peri- and post-operative complications. The National Confidential Enquiry into Peri-Operative Deaths (NCEPOD) has identified night-time operating as contributing to increased morbidity and mortality in this group of patients. In 1987, NCEPOD recommended that such cases should be postponed until normal working hours. Therefore unless there is sufficient clinical justification to proceed, surgery should be delayed until the following day.

Communication with patients and relatives

Effective communication is a two-way process. It enhances patient wellbeing, satisfaction and compliance.

The patient

- *Introduce yourself* and explain what you do and how you fit into the team. Find an appropriate place to take a history and examine the patient
- *Be courteous, respect privacy* and ask the patient if he/she would like a chaperone or relative to be present during the examination
- Spend as much time as you can and *allow the patient to tell their story*
- *Try not to interrupt* or ask leading questions as this may lead you in the wrong direction
- *Always be polite*, even if the patient is not. If you are concerned that a patient is being aggressive or inappropriate, take a member of staff with you, and remember that such behaviour may be a result of their illness
- If the patient does not speak your language *contact an interpreter*, e.g. a relative, member of staff, or service such as 'languageline' that may be able to provide an interpreter over the telephone quickly
- *Don't use jargon.*

Relatives

- *Establish who the relatives are* and whether the patient is happy for you to speak to them
- *Introduce yourself* and explain who you are
- *Find out what they already know* at the beginning of your discussion
- *Try to answer any questions they have accurately*, and if you are not sure say so and explain what you are going to do to find out
- If there are many relatives *ask them to choose one person* for you to speak to, who can then communicate with the rest of the family
- *Try to understand the relatives' concerns*. Coming to hospital is often very stressful/frightening.

Good surgical practice

The General Medical Council has produced a booklet called *Good Surgical Practice* which is designed for all grades of surgeons.[4] It is a document that offers standards by which surgeons can compare their own practice.

---

4 General Medical Council (2002) *Good Surgical Practice*. Royal College of Surgeons, London.

The important points from this document are:

- being available during the on-call period to offer advice and consult
- ensuring that juniors are allowed to perform tasks when it is felt that they are competent to do so
- ensuring that handovers of patients at the end of an on-call period are performed formally
- recognising the need for a second opinion and for senior advice
- ensuring that records are kept in the notes and that these are up to date and legible
- to have regular appraisals
- to participate in regular audit meetings
- informing the consultant on call before taking a patient to theatre
- providing adequate time for patients, and communicating clearly and impartially
- keeping up to date with current guidelines and practices.

Consent

Informed consent

For patients to give their informed consent to surgery, they must make a considered choice about what is in their personal interests. To be able to do this they must receive sufficient information about their illness, the proposed management options and their prognosis.

In the emergency setting, the consent process may be compromised because patients are often in pain, unwell and treatment is urgent. A recent questionnaire study has shown that only 22% of patients undergoing abdominal surgery believed they were adequately informed about side-effects and complications.[5]

Before any procedure a surgeon must impart the following:

- a description of the procedure itself and the probable outcome
- the probability of risks or complications
- alternative treatments that may be available, and their advantages and disadvantages.

When consenting patients, ensure that the patient has understood the points that you have raised. Take into account that English may not be their first language.

5   Kay R and Siriwardena AK (2001) The process of informed consent for urgent abdominal surgery. *J Med Ethics* **27**: 157–61.

Patients aged 18 years or over can refuse life-saving or other treatment provided they are competent (in a legal sense), and fully aware of the possible consequences of their actions.

It is your duty to do whatever is necessary in an emergency to save life or prevent serious disability in patients who are unconscious or unable to give consent. Remember that no adult can give consent on behalf of another adult (aged 18 years or over). It is however important to make reasonable efforts to speak with the next-of-kin in such situations.

Remember to record consent in writing, both on the consent form and in the patient's notes. Also document what has been communicated and in particular any risks or complications. The Department of Health (DOH) has introduced four consent forms:

- *Consent form 1*: patients who can consent themselves
- *Consent form 2*: for parents on behalf of a child
- *Consent form 3*: either patients who can consent themselves or parents on behalf of a child, for a non-general anaesthesia (GA) intervention (optional form)
- *Consent form 4*: patient is an adult unable to consent to an investigation.

Any changes to the consent form must be discussed and signed for by the patient.

Make sure you document right or left side in full (never abbreviate). Digits on the hand should be named, and digits on the foot numbered. Mark the side of the patient.

Mentally impaired patients

Psychiatric illness does not necessarily mean that the patient is incompetent, or unable to give or refuse informed consent.[6]

However, if the patient is deemed incompetent, then the surgeon should, in an emergency, proceed with treatment in the patient's best interests.

Children

The legal age for medical consent is 16 years.

Ordinarily, consent for surgery on young children must always be obtained from a parent or guardian deemed competent to make informed choices regarding the child's best interests.

---

6 A competent adult is a person who is aged over 18 years and has the capacity to make treatment decisions on his or her behalf.

Always assess whether a child below the age of 16 years is capable of understanding the nature and purpose of the proposed treatment. Since the Gillick case a child aged less than 16 years can give consent if he/she demonstrates an understanding of the nature (and risks) of treatment.[7] All children should in any case participate in the decision-making process.

When a competent child up to the age of 18 years refuses treatment when it is considered in their best interest, a parent or court may give consent on behalf of the child. If this situation arises then obtain legal advice from your defence union, or the hospital ethics committee.

If a surgical procedure is clearly in a child's best interests and the parents refuse consent then you should again seek legal advice.

Breaking bad news

Breaking bad news to a patient or family is inherently stressful. Lack of information may be more distressing for a patient than hearing bad news which they may already suspect. A patient who is well informed will adjust better. You must appear competent, honest, and speak clearly.[8] Find a suitable environment for discussion and if possible leave your bleep with a colleague to avoid interruption.

Remember to:

- *review the notes* and *speak to colleagues* before you speak to the patient and family
- *prepare for obvious questions* such as 'what if?' and 'what next?'
- *take somebody with you*, e.g. ward nurse, specialist nurse, who can stay and address any further questions after you have left
- *introduce yourself*, explain what you do, and find out who you're speaking to
- *establish their current level of understanding*
- *allow time* for what you have said to be taken in
- *try to lead up to words* like 'cancer' sensitively, but do not avoid saying them
- *ask if there are any questions*
- *explain how you can be contacted* later if necessary.

When discussing death, people are often concerned that it might be painful. Explain the measures that you will take to alleviate discomfort. Do not give an exact time course for events, as such predictions are often inaccurate.

---

7   *Gillick* v. *West Norfolk and Wisbech Area Health Authority and the Department of Health & Social Security* [1986].
8   Parker PA, Baile WF, de Moor C *et al.* (2001) Breaking bad news about cancer: patients' preferences for communication. *J Clin Oncol* **19**: 2049–56. *See also* Mir NU (2004) Breaking bad news: practical advice for busy doctors. *Hosp Med* **65**: 613–15, and www.breakingbadnews.co.uk (accessed 1 November 2005).

Resuscitation

Discussing resuscitation status may well form part of breaking bad news on the ward. Often it is more appropriate to allow bad news to be digested and to go back later to discuss resuscitation. However, discussion of what happens next may allow an appropriate opportunity to broach the issue. Be clear about what you mean by 'not for resus' and what will still be done, e.g. full active treatment *versus* keeping the patient comfortable.

Dealing with children

Children are often frightened and anxious in hospital, and therefore more difficult to assess. The child may not be able or willing to give you an adequate history. Paediatric nurses and play specialists can be helpful in putting children at ease. Often, parents are very anxious when bringing their child to hospital. Take time to listen to their concerns and reassure them.

When speaking to children remember to:

- *not stand over them* but get down at their level
- *explain what you are doing* and *address them directly*
- *allow them time to answer*, and offer a list of basic responses, e.g. 'is it better, worse or the same?'

During the examination:

- *he/she should be settled and not crying*. It may help to perform the examination after analgesia while a parent holds the child
- you may have to *delay the examination until the child is in a more comfortable environment* (e.g. settled onto the children's ward rather than in a busy emergency department)
- *distraction techniques* may help you to elicit physical signs
- *rectal examination is not routine* in children and may cause distress and loss of trust.

Evidence-based surgery

This is the delivery of optimal surgical treatment based on best current knowledge and evidence.

Surgeons are increasingly required to provide evidence for the decisions that they make. In order to implement evidence-based practice it is necessary for surgeons to assess relevant previous research, and then make a decision as to whether its application is in the best interests of the patient. This decision will also depend on the wishes of the patient (e.g. a patient may want to have a shortened but better quality of life rather than increased longevity by having adjuvant chemotherapy).

Randomised controlled trials and meta-analyses represent the highest form of evidence. The majority of surgical practice is evidence based, but the proportion from randomised controlled trials remains small. There are many reasons for this:

- it is not ethical to perform placebo operations
- operator experience may have an important impact on the results of any procedure and the incidence of complications
- blinding of patients is extremely difficult or impossible, particularly if the operations that are being compared result in different types of wounds (e.g. laparoscopic versus open surgery)
- surgical trials are liable to be extremely expensive, and funding for them is especially difficult.

Many have argued that there needs to be an increase in randomised trials in surgery, despite the problems highlighted above. However, alternative research designs may be the answer, for instance trials that incorporate patient preference.

When trying to implement evidence-based surgery (EBS) in the acute setting, follow the steps shown in Figure 1.1.

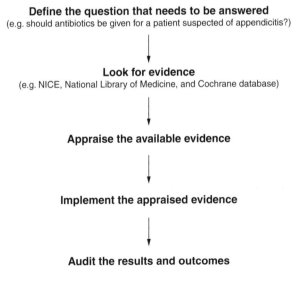

Define the question that needs to be answered
(e.g. should antibiotics be given for a patient suspected of appendicitis?)

Look for evidence
(e.g. NICE, National Library of Medicine, and Cochrane database)

Appraise the available evidence

Implement the appraised evidence

Audit the results and outcomes

Figure 1.1   Steps in implementing evidence-based surgery.

Assessment of clinical guidelines[9]

Clinical guidelines are 'systematically developed statements to assist practitioner and patients' decisions about appropriate health care for specific clinical circumstances'.[10]

They are issued as a means of improving quality of healthcare, and may be used as a point of reference to compare clinicians' practices. However, guidelines are often produced by appraising evidence from randomised controlled trials, and therefore may not be appropriate for a particular clinical scenario. Guideline recommendations can be incorrect, inhibit clinicians' freedom of choice and also stifle research in an area of interest. There may also be legal considerations to take into account.

Nevertheless in the UK the importance of clinical practice guidelines is growing, and they are an integral part of improving quality of healthcare provision.

For an index of current UK guidelines and those that are in progress visit: http://libraries.nelh.nhs.uk/guidelinesFinder/.

Blood-borne diseases/universal precautions

The three blood-borne viruses that are most important to surgeons are *HIV*, *hepatitis B*, and *hepatitis C*.

HIV

In certain parts of the world this is a major problem. Transmission of HIV in the hospital is a relatively rare event. The highest risk is to nurses and laboratory personnel. Furthermore the rate of HIV transmission following a needlestick injury is about 0.3%. If you receive a needlestick injury remember to report it and follow your hospital's protocol.

Hepatitis B

All clinicians should be vaccinated against this virus. Ensure that you have had a recent positive antibody titre. Your occupational health department will normally check immunity as a prerequisite to employment.

---

9   Andrews EJ and Redmond HP (2004) A review of clinical guidelines. *Br J Surg* 91: 956–64.
10 Field MJ and Lohr KN (eds) (1990) *Clinical Practice Guidelines: directions for a new program, Institute of Medicine*. National Academy Press, Washington, DC.

Hepatitis C

This is now a major concern. The rate of hepatitis C transmission following a needlestick injury can be up to 3%. Unlike HIV there is no effective post-exposure prophylaxis. There is a much higher chance of developing chronic hepatitis after hepatitis C infection compared to hepatitis B.

When carrying out procedures the surgeon should adopt a policy of 'universal precautions':

- *wear gloves* when handling human tissue and when performing phlebotomy
- *wear masks, gowns and protective eyewear* when carrying out any procedures
- *wash hands thoroughly* immediately after any exposure to bodily fluids
- *take special precaution when handling instruments and needles/scalpels*
- *dispose of sharp items in designated sharps' bins* immediately after use.

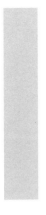

Chapter 2

Assessment of the general surgical patient

Assessment of the general surgical patient

Perform the following in this order.

1 *Resuscitation and analgesia*
2 *History*
3 *Examination*
4 *Special investigations*
5 *Documentation.*

Resuscitation and analgesia

All patients should have a short but immediate assessment to determine the need for resuscitation (ABC):

- *A (airway)*: speak to the patient. If they can talk their airway is patent. If there is an airway concern call an anaesthetist
- *B (breathing)*: examine the chest, check O_2 saturations and respiratory rate. Give oxygen if needed
- *C (circulation)*: measure blood pressure and pulse. Check peripheral perfusion (capillary refill). Establish intravenous access and administer crystalloid or colloid fluid as necessary.

Assess the need for pain relief and administer analgesia (*see* 'Analgesia', page 26).

History

A good history will establish the diagnosis in the majority of cases.

If the patient is unwell (especially in the trauma setting) you may only have time for an AMPLE history:

- *A*: allergies
- *M*: medications
- *P*: PMH (previous medical history), pregnancy
- *L*: last meal
- *E*: events leading to admission.

If the patient is stable a full history should be taken:

- *PC: presenting complaint* – one sentence to describe why the patient came to hospital, e.g. right iliac fossa pain
- *HPC: history of the presenting complaint* – full details of the history of the main complaint should be sought

- *PMH: previous medical history* – asthma, epilepsy, diabetes mellitus, myocardial infarction (MI), TB, rheumatic fever, angina, hypertension, stroke and any previous admissions/surgery
- *DH: drug history* – all medication and nature of any allergies, e.g. rash/anaphylaxis
- *SE: systems enquiry* – cardiovascular, respiratory, gastrointestinal and neurological:
    - is the patient fit for surgery/anaesthesia?
    - what is the patient's usual level of activity?
- *FH: family history* – any relevant family history of illness
- *SOH: social and occupational history* – smoking/alcohol/drug use.

General examination

- *General appearance*: e.g. well, alert, sitting up in bed
- *Observations*: pulse, blood pressure, temperature, respiratory rate (often omitted and a good early indicator if unwell)
- *Peripheries*: warm/cool, capillary refill
- *Jugular venous pressure (JVP)* + look for signs of *dehydration*[1]
- Look for *jaundice, anaemia, cyanosis, clubbing, oedema, lymphadenopathy (JACCOL)*
- *Mini-mental test score* or *GCS (Glasgow Coma Scale)* if confused or consciousness level is impaired.

Then:

- examine the site of interest, e.g. abdomen, lower limbs.

Special investigations

Before you request any investigation think about what you are looking for and how it will influence management.

For all patients

1 *Check BM*: diabetes can present with abdominal pain, as well as complicate surgical illness and recovery

---

1 Lethargy, confusion, dry mucous membranes, sunken eyes, decreased skin turgor and low urine output.

2 *Urine dipstick*: usually positive in the presence of a urinary tract infection (UTI). It may be positive if there is an inflammatory process adjacent to the renal tract such as appendicitis. β-*HCG* (human chorionic gonadotrophin) should be checked in all females of child-bearing age.

Blood tests

1 *Full blood count (FBC)*: high or very low white cell count occurs in sepsis; low haemoglobin (Hb)/haematocrit may reflect blood loss; low platelets in bleeding/disseminated intravascular coagulation (DIC)
2 *Urea and electrolytes (U&Es)*: baseline renal function, urea may be elevated out of proportion to creatinine in dehydration. Electrolyte disturbances can occur in vomiting/diarrhoea/third-space losses
3 *C-reactive protein (CRP)*: inflammatory marker produced by the liver
4 *Amylase*: >1000 U/l for diagnosis of acute pancreatitis, but may be normal in acute on chronic, and can be high in other conditions, e.g. perforated viscus
5 *Liver function tests (LFTs)*: hepatobiliary disease, suspicion of metastatic disease, jaundice
6 *Clotting*: pre-operative; especially if liver disease or prior use of anticoagulants
7 *Group and save*: +/– cross-match blood
8 *Arterial blood gas*: information about gas exchange and acid–base balance.

Radiological investigations

1 *Erect CXR*: e.g. free air under diaphragm may be seen in perforated viscus
2 *Supine abdominal X-ray (AXR)*: e.g. obstruction, volvulus, may see abdominal aortic aneurysm (AAA)
3 *Ultrasound scan (USS)*: very useful, simple, used for evaluation of a mass, examination of the liver/biliary tree/gallbladder/kidneys/ovaries/uterus
4 *CT*: extremely useful for a wide range of pathologies
5 *Instant enema*: useful to establish level of large bowel obstruction
6 *Intravenous urogram (IVU)*: e.g. renal stones/obstructed renal tract.

Documentation

● A *clearly written, dated and signed account* in the medical notes is a legal requirement and your only defence if there is a problem later. If you have requested a test you should make sure the results are checked and documented.

Fluid balance

Total body water:

> = 60% in males, 55% in females and 75% in a child
> = 45 l in a 70 kg male.

Of the total body water (in a 70 kg male) two-thirds is intracellular (30 l) and one-third is extracellular (15 l) – *see* Figure 2.1.

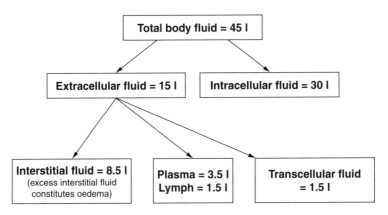

Figure 2.1   Body fluid compartments.

Extracellular fluid includes intravascular and extravascular compartments separated by the capillary membrane (distribution of fluid is governed by Starling's hypothesis[2]). The transcellular fluid compartment includes bone, synovial fluid, gastrointestinal luminal fluid, cerebrospinal fluid (CSF) and the aqueous humor of the eye. Fluid sequestered within this compartment accounts for 'third space' losses.

The ionic composition of each fluid compartment is shown in Table 2.1.

Table 2.1   The ionic composition (mmol/l) of different fluid compartments

	Plasma	*Interstitial fluid*	*Intracellular fluid*
Na^+	140	145	10
K^+	4	4	160
Ca^{2+}	2	2	0
Cl^-	100	115	3
HCO_3	28	30	10

---

2   This governs the relationship between intra and extraluminal hydrostatic/oncotic pressures with fluid passage across the capillary membrane.

Assessing fluid balance status

A 'dry' patient may have:

- thirst
- cool peripheries with increased capillary refill time
- dry tongue
- reduced skin turgor
- tachycardia
- confusion
- hypotension
- sunken eyes
- high specific gravity on urine dipstick
- increased serum urea
- increased haematocrit.

Monitoring fluid balance

- Catheterisation + hourly urine volumes (maintain urine output of at least 0.5 ml/kg/h[3])
- An accurate fluid balance chart
- Daily weights may be helpful
- Central venous pressure (CVP) response to a fluid challenge.

Fluid replacement

To achieve adequate fluid balance, losses (including insensible losses such as sweat, and fluid lost through respiration) must be replaced in addition to normal maintenance needs. The average daily water requirements for an adult are 30–35 ml/kg + 500 ml/day/degree of pyrexia (above 37°C). Adult electrolyte requirements are 1 mmol/kg each of Na^+, K^+ and Cl^-.[4]

Normal fluid requirements for children depend on weight:

- *<10 kg*: 100 ml/kg/day
- *10–20 kg*: 1 l + 50 ml/kg/day
- *>20 kg*: 1.5 l + 25 ml/kg/day.

---

3   For children aim for 1 ml/kg/h.
4   A suitable regime of maintenance fluid for a 70 kg adult is 1 l normal saline and 2 l 5% dextrose with 20 mmol KCl per litre, over 24 h.

Crystalloids

Crystalloids are electrolyte solutions in water. Up to 40 mmol KCl can be added to each litre on the ward. Table 2.2 shows the concentrations of electrolytes in commonly prescribed crystalloids.

Table 2.2   Concentrations (mmol/l) of electrolytes in commonly used crystalloids

	Na^+	K^+	HCO_3	Cl^-	Ca^{2+}
0.9% Normal saline	154	–	–	154	–
Hartmann's solution	131	5	29	111	2
Dextrose saline	30	–	–	30	–
5% Dextrose	–	–	–	–	–

Colloids

Colloids contain higher molecular weight molecules than crystalloids and will therefore remain longer in the intravascular compartment. They are used as a short-term measure to expand plasma volume and improve blood pressure. However, the use of colloids may prolong tissue oedema.

Types of colloid include:

● gelatins, e.g. Gelofusine, Haemaccel
● dextrans, e.g. Hespan, dextran
● albumin, e.g. human albumin solution (HAS).

Blood transfusion

Blood transfusion will:

- replace intravascular volume
- increase oxygen-carrying capacity (avoiding anaerobic metabolism and subsequent build-up of oxygen debt).[5]

A unit of blood is 350 ml and should increase Hb by approximately 1 g/dl.

When to transfuse?

Hb < 8 g/dl is often used as a trigger for transfusion. However it has been shown that transfusion at a Hb of 7 g/dl and a maintenace range of 7–9 g/dl is either equivalent, or in some patient groups (particularly those <55 years old) superior to, maintaining a Hb >10 g/dl.[6]

A liberal transfusion policy can lead to worsening patient outcomes including higher mortality, longer hospital stay and increased rates of organ dysfunction.[7] This may be due to exposure to allogenic leucocytes. The subsequent immunological response leads to an increased risk of infection and tumour recurrence.[8]

Critical illness itself, irrespective of blood loss, is associated with a fall in Hb (related to a reduction in the production of erythropoietin and changes in iron metabolism). A lower Hb/haematocrit may be beneficial in terms of microcirculation perfusion.

Decisions concerning transfusion should be tailored to physiological need rather than a particular Hb value. For any patient consider the pre-operative Hb, cardiovascular and respiratory status (for example a patient with chronic lung or cardiac disease may need to be transfused to a higher level).

---

5 Transfused blood has reduced O_2-carrying capacity as it is depleted in 2,3-diphosphoglycerate (2,3-DPG) after 10 days' storage (*see* oxygen dissociation curve – Chapter 3, page 45).
6 Herbert PC (1998) Transfusion requirements in critical care (TRICC): a multicentre, randomized, controlled clinical study. Transfusion Requirements in Critical Care Investigators and the Canadian Critical Care Trials Group. *Br J Anaesth* **81** (Suppl 1): 25–33.
7   Vincent JL, Baron JF, Gattinoni L *et al.* (2002) Anemia and blood transfusions in the critically ill: an epidemiological, observational study. *JAMA* **288**: 1499–507.
8   Bordin JO, Heddle NM and Bujchman MA (1994) Biologic effects of leucocytes present in transfused cellular blood products. *Blood* **84**: 1703–21.

Problems associated with blood transfusion

- Risk of *bacterial contamination*. Blood is screened for certain viral infections including HIV, hepatitis B and C, and syphilis
- Risk of *incompatibility*
- Risk of *fluid overload*. Consider giving furosemide with blood transfusion in the elderly and those with cardiovascular disease
- Blood that has been stored for more than 2 days has *no effective platelets*. There is also a reduced oxygen-carrying capacity and reduced lifespan in the circulation
- *Immune suppression*. Transfusion of leucodepleted blood should not be limited by concerns of increased tumour recurrence or peri-operative infection[9]
- *Hypothermia*, which also has an adverse effect on platelet aggregation. Warm blood before transfusion
- *Prions*: unknown risk.

Massive blood transfusion

Massive blood transfusion is defined as transfusion of the patient's total blood volume within 24 h.

Effects of massive transfusion include:

- dilution of platelets and clotting factors
- hypocalcaemia
- hyperkalaemia
- acidosis
- acute respiratory distress syndrome (ARDS)
- disseminated intravascular coagulation (DIC)
- jaundice.

Incompatibility

Incompatibility reactions vary in severity.

- It is common to see a *mild increase in temperature* following blood transfusion due to host antibodies to donor white blood cells. If this occurs the rate of infusion should be slowed and paracetamol given

---

9 SIGN (Scottish Intercollegiate Guideline Network) *Guidance 54 on Perioperative Blood Transfusion for Elective Surgery*, 2001 www.sign.ac.uk (accessed 2 November 2005).

- ABO incompatibility results in an *acute haemolytic reaction*. It occurs very rapidly after as little as 5 ml of blood transfusion. It manifests as itching, chest pain, agitation and a rapid rise in temperature to >40°C. If this occurs the transfusion should be stopped immediately. Check the patient's identity and compare with the blood transfusion. Inform the blood bank and send samples of the patient and donor blood to them
- A *delayed haemolytic reaction* occurs up to 10 days following transfusion in 1 in 500 transfusions, resulting in fever, anaemia, jaundice and hemoglobinuria
- *Anaphylaxis* can also occur following blood transfusion. If this occurs stop the transfusion, give oxygen, chlorpheniramine i.v., and adrenaline as necessary
- *TRALI (transfusion-related acute lung injury)* can occur due to incompatibility between donor antibodies and recipient white blood cells. It manifests as fever, cough, shortness of breath and lung infiltrates on CXR.

Pre-operative group and save

Most hospitals publish guidelines on who should have a 'group and save' pre-operatively, and the number of units that should be cross-matched for a particular procedure.

In order to minimise errors when taking a sample, blood should be taken from only one patient at a time. Check their name, date of birth and wristband, and label the bottle at the bedside.

It takes approximately 10 min to group a blood sample and up to 40 min for a full cross-match. If there is insufficient time O negative blood is the universal donor.

Other blood products and their uses[10]

- *Platelets*: these are rarely needed. Give if the platelet count is <50×10^9/l and the patient is bleeding, or an invasive procedure is about to be performed. Platelets need to be ABO compatible
- *Fresh frozen plasma (FFP)*: fresh frozen plasma contains all clotting factors; 1 unit of FFP should be given with every 4 units of blood transfused. It can also be used to reverse a high international normalised ratio (INR) in patients taking warfarin before emergency surgery and in DIC

---

10 No authors listed (1994) Practice parameter for the use of fresh-frozen plasma, cryoprecipitate, and platelets. Fresh-Frozen Plasma, Cryoprecipitate, and Platelets Administration Practice Guidelines Development Task Force of the College of American Pathologists. *JAMA* **271**: 777–81.

- *Cryoprecipitate*: this is formed by slow thawing of FFP and is rich in von Willebrand factor (vWF), factor VIII and fibrinogen, and is therefore used in DIC
- *Individual clotting factors*: e.g. factor VIII are available
- *Human albumin solution (HAS)*: this has no proven benefit over synthetic colloids in blood volume expansion. The only indication for the use of HAS is diuretic-resistant oedema in hyponatraemic patients.

Patients who refuse transfusion

Any patient can legally refuse a blood transfusion. Enquire if they would accept autologous transfusion instead, e.g. donating their own blood pre-operatively, or the use of a cell saver device during surgery.

Analgesia

The provision of adequate analgesia in the emergency setting is essential. Relieving pain will allow the patient to give a better history, tolerate clinical examination and any subsequent investigations/treatment.[11] There is evidence that patients often receive inadequate analgesia either from their GP or in the accident and emergency department.

The amount and type of analgesia must be tailored to the individual's needs.

Systemic analgesia

A useful means of ensuring adequate analgesia is to prescribe a range of analgesics with different strengths and mechanisms of action, the so-called analgesia 'ladder' (*see* Figure 2.2). The strength of analgesia given can be increased until the patient is comfortable. In addition, this system allows synergistic action between different groups of analgesics.

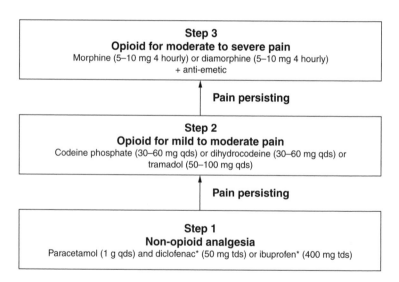

Step 3
Opioid for moderate to severe pain
Morphine (5–10 mg 4 hourly) or diamorphine (5–10 mg 4 hourly)
+ anti-emetic

↑
Pain persisting

Step 2
Opioid for mild to moderate pain
Codeine phosphate (30–60 mg qds) or dihydrocodeine (30–60 mg qds) or
tramadol (50–100 mg qds)

↑
Pain persisting

Step 1
Non-opioid analgesia
Paracetamol (1 g qds) and diclofenac* (50 mg tds) or ibuprofen* (400 mg tds)

* Caution in patients with renal impairment, peptic ulcer disease and asthma.

Figure 2.2   The analgesia ladder (adult doses given).

---

11 Narcotic analgesia does not cause adverse outcomes or delays in diagnosis in the emergency setting. *See* McHale PM and LoVecchio F (2001) Narcotic analgesia in the acute abdomen – a review of prospective trials. *Eur J Emerg Med* 8: 131–6.

Note:

1 patients in severe discomfort should be given an opiate intravenously as first-line analgesia, and this should be titrated until pain is adequately controlled
2 adequacy of pain relief should be reviewed regularly.

Patient-controlled analgesia (PCA)

This is a useful means of giving strong opiate analgesia in the acute setting. Patients control the amount of analgesia they receive. The standard regimen is a bolus of 1 mg of morphine given with a 5 min lockout time before another dose can be delivered. Consequently, dosing is automatically tailored to the individual's need. PCA is at least as effective as nurse-delivered analgesia and may be just as effective in the emergency setting.[12]

Local anaesthesia

Table 2.3 shows safe doses in adults.[13]

Table 2.3 Safe doses of local anaesthetics in adults

	Plain	*With adrenaline*[14]
Lignocaine/lidocaine	3 mg/kg	7 mg/kg
Bupivacaine	2 mg/kg	3 mg/kg

Local anaesthetic (LA) agents have a limited role in the acute general surgical patient. They are useful for:

- *minor procedures* in the accident and emergency department, e.g. cleaning, exploring, suturing small superficial wounds, draining perianal haematoma
- *local analgesic blocks*, e.g. at the site of rib fractures
- *to aid cannulation* in children, e.g. topical application of local anaesthetic cream.

---

12 Evans E, Turley N, Robinson N and Clancy M (2005) Randomised controlled trial of patient controlled analgesia compared with nurse delivered analgesia in an emergency department. *Emerg Med J* 22: 25–9.
13 To calculate dose remember: 100% lignocaine = 1000 g in 1000 ml, 1% is 10 g (or 10 000 mg) in 1000 ml, therefore 1 ml of 1% is equivalent to 10 mg.
14 Adrenaline with LA has some advantages. By causing vasoconstriction it may help with control of bleeding, increase the duration of action, and reduce systemic absorption. Adrenaline should never be used in the extremities.

Caution should be taken in the presence of overt infection or pus because:

- injection of local anaesthetic may disseminate infection into deeper tissues
- local anaesthesia will not work as well.[15]

Symptoms of LA toxicity include: light-headedness, tinnitus, tongue numbness, visual disturbances, muscle twitching, convulsions and loss of consciousness.

Epidural anaesthesia

This is particularly useful for the post-operative patient, but may also be of use in patients who have chest trauma (e.g. rib injuries, restricting breathing). There is less sedation, respiratory depression and better ambulation compared to narcotics.

---

15 Local anaesthetic agents dissociate poorly in the acidic environment that exists within infected tissue.

Antibiotics and emergency general surgery

The goal of antibiotic therapy is to reduce the number of bacteria-invading tissues.

In this respect antibiotics can be either *bacteriostatic* (preventing growth and multiplication) or *bactericidal* (kill bacteria).

Antibiotics are often overprescribed and can contribute to toxicity, emergence of resistant strains and superinfection by other organisms (e.g. *Candida* and *C. difficile*).

Remember, if you have any doubts about which antibiotic to use (if any), especially if the patient has an allergy, then discuss this with your microbiologist. They are usually very helpful and keen to get involved.

Antibiotic prophylaxis

Antibiotic prophylaxis should ideally be given within 1 h of starting the procedure. Appropriate use has been shown to lower the incidence of post-operative wound infection. It is not necessary to repeat the dosage during surgery unless there is either contamination or more than 1 l of blood loss, since there is evidence that clearance of antibiotics is slower in patients undergoing surgery.[16] After surgery there is usually no additional benefit from administering further doses, except when there is heavy contamination.

Which operations should have antibiotic prophylaxis?

Antibiotic prophylaxis is recommended for the following emergency operations:

- colorectal surgery
- appendicectomy
- small bowel and gastroduodenal surgery
- hernia surgery (involving use of a mesh)
- lower limb revascularisation or amputation
- open biliary surgery.

In particular the following operations do not normally need prophylaxis:

- laparoscopic cholecystectomy
- hernia repair without mesh.

---

16 Van Dijk-van Dam MS, Moll FL, de Letter JA, Langemeijer JJ and Kuks PF (1996) The myth of the second prophylactic antibiotic dose in aortoiliac reconstructions. *Eur J Vasc Endovasc Surg* 12: 428–30.

Nosocomial infections[17]

These are otherwise known as hospital-acquired infections. They cost hospitals in the UK over a billion pounds per annum and in surgical patients commonly affect the chest, urinary tract, bloodstream and wounds.

Wound infections

Table 2.4 offers a simplistic guide to treatment of surgical site infections (SSIs).[18] Classic signs are *tumour* (swelling), *dolor* (pain), *rubor* (redness) and *calor* (heat). The following are risk factors for the development of a SSI:

- type of surgery (e.g. colorectal > cholecystectomy)
- length of wound
- poor blood supply or tension in the wound
- poor surgical technique
- age
- diabetes mellitus
- immunocompromise
- length of hospital stay.

Table 2.4   Types of surgical site infections, organisms responsible and suggested antibiotics

	Organism	Antibiotic
General wound infections	Staphylococcus aureus	Flucloxacillin, ciprofloxacin, clindamycin
	Beta-haemolytic Streptococcus	Penicillins, ciprofloxacin, clindamycin
Operations above the waist: upper gastrointestinal tract	Enteric Gram-negative bacilli	Cefuroxime, co-amoxiclav, gentamicin
Operations below the waist: colorectal	Enteric Gram-negative bacilli	Cefuroxime, co-amoxiclav, gentamicin
	Anaerobes	Metronidazole, co-amoxiclav
Procedures involving insertion of prosthetic material	Coagulase-negative Staphylococcus	Vancomycin + removal of prosthetic material (60–80% methicillin resistant)

17 Leaper D (2004) Nosocomial infection. *Br J Surg* **91**: 526–7.
18 A surgical site infection (SSI) is a post-operative complication occurring within 30 days of a surgical procedure (usually occurring within a week post-operatively). Prevalence is roughly 10% but this is higher for acute surgery. The National Institute for Clinical Excellence (NICE) is currently working on guidelines for managing SSIs.

Wound dehiscence

Dehiscence occurs when part or all of the operative wound is disrupted. Occasionally it leads to evisceration of bowel. It occurs most commonly about one week after surgery.

Risk factors for wound dehiscence include:

- poor surgical technique
- tension in wound
- poor blood supply to the wound
- diabetes mellitus
- obesity
- high intra-abdominal compartment pressure
- malnutrition
- wound infection
- coughing (either chronic or associated with a chest infection).

Leakage of serosanguinous fluid from the wound may precede dehiscence.

Evisceration must be treated immediately and involves placing warm wet packs over the wound, and closing the wound in theatre. Before closing it is important to check the integrity of any intra-abdominal anastomoses.

MRSA (methicillin-resistant *Staphylococcus aureus*)

MRSA causes considerable morbidity and mortality in the UK. Carriers can be identified in most cases by nasal swabbing. Risk factors for infection are:

- age
- length of hospital stay
- chronic illness (e.g. diabetes)
- prolonged antibiotic therapy
- open wounds
- presence of an indwelling device (e.g. catheter or central line).

Effective control measures for MRSA include:

- screening of patients
- handwashing
- use of mupirocin
- isolation of carriers and infected patients
- body cleansing with povidone iodine.

Intravenous vancomycin is the drug of choice for infection (a bactericidal glycopeptide). Oral administration is not commonly used because it is poorly absorbed from the gastrointestinal (GI) tract. Ensure serum levels are performed. Teicoplanin may be used as an alternative to vancomycin.[19] Other agents should be used in combination and include clindamycin and rifampicin. Such regimens should be discussed with the microbiologists.

---

19 A newer antibiotic, linezolid, may be superior to vancomycin in treating MRSA infection. *See* Weigelt J, Kaafarani HM, Itani KM and Swanson RN (2004) Linezolid eradicates MRSA better than vancomycin from surgical-site infections. *Am J Surg* **188**: 760–6.

Deep venous thrombosis prophylaxis

Prevalence

Without antithrombotic prophylaxis 8–15% of patients develop deep venous thrombosis (DVT) after major general surgery, and 36–60% after surgery for hip fracture.

Pathogenesis

The factors that promote venous thrombosis are known as *Virchow's triad*:

- *reduction of blood flow*: stasis from being in a supine position during surgery
- *hypercoagulability*: decreased clearance of procoagulant factors
- *abnormalities in the vessel wall*: exarcerbated by vasodilation during anaesthesia.

Risk factors for DVT

- *Increasing age*
- *Pregnancy*
- *Malignancy*
- *Previous history of DVT*
- *Varicose veins*
- *Obesity*
- *Immobility*
- *Hypercoagulable state* (protein C/protein S deficiency, factor V Leiden mutation).

Every acute surgical admission should be started on DVT prophylaxis (subcutaneous heparin or low-molecular-weight heparin, e.g. tinzaparin 3500 units od s.c.) unless there are contraindications.

Absolute contraindications to DVT prophylaxis

- *Bleeding*
- *Severe bleeding diathesis*
- *Platelet count <20 000/μl.*

Relative contraindications to DVT prophylaxis

- *Moderate bleeding diathesis*
- *Recent trauma*
- *Infective endocarditis*
- *Malignant hypertension.*

TED stockings and *early ambulation* are two important non-pharmacological measures for reducing the risk of DVT.

Preparing the patient for theatre

Pre-operative measures are important to optimise the patient's clinical status prior to theatre and thereby reduce the chance of peri-operative complications. Fluid balance, electrolyte, metabolic and haematological disturbances should be corrected prior to surgery wherever possible.

Routine measures

- Ensure the patient is nil by mouth
- Ensure adequate intravenous access
- Prescribe appropriate intravenous fluids
- Prescribe adequate analgesia
- Prescribe appropriate DVT prophylaxis
- Mark side-specific pathology with an indelible skin marker
- Obtain informed consent for the proposed surgical intervention.

Additional measures

Additional measures may include:

- blood tests (e.g. electrolytes)
- cross-match blood if necessary
- ECG and CXR
- supplemental oxygen
- antibiotics
- nasogastric tube insertion to decompress the stomach
- urinary catheterisation to monitor urine output
- central venous line insertion to monitor central venous pressure.

Inform

- The on-call anaesthetist
- Theatres
- On-call radiographer if required.

Preparing special patient groups for theatre

Patients with diabetes

Added risks

- Hypoglycaemia
- Ketoacidosis
- Impaired wound healing
- Wound infection
- Cardiovascular complications.

Management

- Tight glycaemic control reduces the risk of post-operative complications. Stop regular hypoglycaemic agents
- Patients with non-insulin-dependent diabetes (NIDDM) who are undergoing a minor procedure where a protracted post-operative recovery time is not anticipated can often be managed with regular BM measurements and no sliding scale
- Patients with insulin-dependent diabetes (IDDM) or non-insulin-dependent diabetes who are undergoing a major procedure should be managed with an i.v. insulin sliding scale
- If in doubt discuss with the anaesthetist.

Jaundiced patients

Added risks

- Impaired wound healing
- Wound infection
- Clotting abnormalities/bleeding
- Hepatic and renal impairment.

Management

Correct clotting abnormalities (10 mg vitamin K i.v. repeated every 24 h. For urgent correction give fresh frozen plasma). Ensure the patient is adequately hydrated, catheterised and urine output closely monitored. The patient will need daily U&Es post-operatively.

Patients on steroids

Added risks

- Adrenal suppression resulting in inability to mount an adequate 'stress response'
- Impaired wound healing
- Wound infection
- Haematoma
- Stress ulceration.

Management

The patient may require additional steroid cover during the peri-operative period (e.g. in major surgery 100 mg hydrocortisone i.v. at induction, then 6-hourly for the next 48 h. Reduce to pre-operative dose over next 5–7 days).

Patients on warfarin

Added risks

- Bleeding.

Management

Management will depend on the reason for anticoagulation. Stop warfarin. Correct clotting abnormality (2 mg vitamin K i.v.; for urgent correction give fresh frozen plasma). Low-dose vitamin K temporarily reverses anticoagulant effect of warfarin and will have little effect on the efficacy of warfarin when restarted post-operatively. The patient may require intravenous heparin as a substitute for warfarin (e.g. if they have a mechanical heart valve). This should be stopped 6 h prior to surgery and requires monitoring of the activated partial thromboplastin time (APTT). If in doubt seek advice from a haematologist.

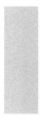

Chapter 3
Critical care

Shock

Shock is defined as *inadequate organ perfusion and tissue oxygenation*. Shock can be classified according to its cause:

- hypovolaemic
- septic
- anaphylactic
- cardiogenic
- neurogenic.

Hypovolaemic shock

This is due to loss of intravascular volume (blood loss or severe dehydration). Loss of circulating volume results in activation of the sympathetic nervous system. There is an increase in heart rate and vasoconstriction of skin, muscle, and GI beds in order to direct blood to vital organs, i.e. heart, brain.

As a result of vasoconstriction of the renal and splanchnic circulation, renal failure, GI sloughing and GI haemorrhage can occur. With more severe shock, reduced perfusion of the brain results in confusion and aggression. Initially there is a respiratory alkalosis due to hyperventilation. Subsequently a metabolic acidosis occurs due to inadequate tissue perfusion and anaerobic metabolism. This is detrimental to cardiac function and the inotropic effect of circulating catecholamines.

In the initial stages of hypovolaemic shock auto-transfusion of up to 1 l of fluid/h occurs from interstitial spaces back into circulation (*see* 'Fluid balance', page 19). Antidiuretic hormone (ADH) secreted from the posterior pituitary acts to increase fluid reabsorption by the kidneys, as well as acting as a vasoconstrictor. Activation of the renin–angiotensin system leads to further vasoconstriction (angiotensin) and fluid reabsorption (aldosterone).

In early shock, a hypercoagulable state develops as thromboxane A_2 from ischaemic tissue leads to aggregation of platelets and extensive microembolic events. This is superseded by fibrinolysis.

Table 3.1 shows the classification of hypovolaemic shock.

Treatment of hypovolaemic shock

- *Control of haemorrhage*
- *Restoration of circulating volume*: classes 1 and 2 shock may be treated with crystalloid/colloid replacement, while classes 3 and 4 will require blood transfusion. Give a fluid challenge of 1–2 l for adults and 20 ml/kg for children initially. A rapid correction in blood pressure/pulse suggests blood loss is probably <20%. If there is only a transient response, resuscitation is

either inadequate or losses are ongoing. No response suggests a need for immediate surgical intervention.

Table 3.1 Classification of hypovolaemic shock

Class	Blood loss	Pulse (per min)	Blood pressure	Urine output (ml/h)	Respiratory rate (per min)	Conscious state
I	<15% (0–750 ml)	60–100	No change	>30	<20	No change
II	15–30% (750–1500 ml)	>100	Pulse pressure reduced	20–30	20–30	Anxious
III	30–40% (1500–2000 ml)	>120	↓	5–15	30–40	Confused
IV	>40% (>2000 ml)	>140	↓↓	Anuria	>40	Lethargic

Septic shock

Septic shock is severe sepsis with hypoperfusion (indicated by a raised serum lactate and metabolic acidosis). *See* page 43.

Anaphylactic shock

Anaphylactic shock is a type I hypersensitivity reaction mediated by immunoglobulin E (IgE). In hospital this is usually due to drugs, blood transfusion or radiological contrast. It presents with a widespread urticarial rash, bronchospasm resulting in wheeze, tachycardia, hypotension and soft tissue oedema due to vasodilatation and capillary leak.

Treatment

1 *Stop the cause* if known
2 *Manage the airway* (call an anaesthetist) + give *100% O_2*
3 Get *i.v. access* and give *fluids*
4 Give *adrenaline* (1 ml of 1 in 1000 given intramuscularly)
5 Give *chlorpheniramine* 10 mg + *hydrocortisone* 100 mg
6 Consider *bronchodilators*.

Cardiogenic shock

Cardiogenic shock occurs due to pump failure. Classically it occurs after a myocardial infarction or pulmonary embolus. Occasionally cardiogenic shock can result from blunt cardiac injury or cardiac tamponade. Seek urgent critical care review.

Neurogenic shock

Neurogenic shock can occur after spinal cord injury. There is a disruption of autonomic nervous system (sympathetic) control over vasoconstriction. This results in a decrease in peripheral vascular resistance and blood pressure, with an absence of reflex tachycardia or an associated inappropriate bradycardia. There may also be loss of temperature control. Exclude other causes of hypotension. Management involves close monitoring, careful fluid management and inotropic support.

Systemic inflammatory response syndrome (SIRS) and sepsis

SIRS is characterised by two or more of the following:

- temperature of >38°C or <36°C
- heart rate >90 beats/min
- respiratory rate (RR) >20/min
- WBC >12 or <4 ×10^9/l.

SIRS may occur as a result of infection or inflammation (for example pancreatitis, trauma or burns). SIRS is mediated by acute phase cytokines (tumour necrosis factor (TNF)-α, interleukin (Il)-1, Il-2, Il-8, Il-10, and in particular Il-6), which have a generalised effect distant to the site of the initial insult. Leucocytes adhere to endothelial cells via adhesion molecules (E-selectin, P-selectin, intercellular adhesion molecule (ICAM)-1) leading to changes in vascular permeability and oedema. Adult respiratory distress syndrome (ARDS) can occur. GI bacterial translocation is thought to be important in SIRS and the development of MODS (multi-organ dysfunction syndrome).

Sepsis is SIRS where an infective organism has been identified as the cause.

Treatment of sepsis[1]

- *Resuscitate* the patient[2]
- *Find the source of sepsis*: take cultures (blood cultures, mid-stream urine (MSU), wound swab, other, e.g. pleural fluid) *before* starting empirical broad-spectrum antibiotics (discuss with the microbiologists if necessary). The only exception to this rule is bacterial meningitis/meningococcal septicaemia when antibiotics should be given as soon as the diagnosis is suspected
- *Drain any abscesses/collections*
- Consider *discussion with high-dependency unit (HDU)/intensive therapy unit (ITU)*.

---

1 Delinger RP, Carlet JM, Masur H *et al.* (2004) Surviving Sepsis Campaign guidelines for management of severe sepsis and septic shock. *Intensive Care Med* 30: 536–55.

2 'Early goal-directed therapy' is a term used to describe targets for resuscitation, which, if achieved within 6 h, can reduce mortality. These targets include CVP 8–12 mmHg, mean arterial pressure >65 mmHg, urine output >0.5 ml/kg/h, central or mixed oxygen saturation >70%. From Rivers E, Nguyen B, Harstad S *et al.* (2001) Early goal directed therapy in the treatment of severe sepsis and septic shock. *N Engl J Med* 345: 1368–77.

Critical care management of severe sepsis may include:

- *vasopressors* (usually noradrenaline) to combat vasodilatation and maintain adequate blood pressure and perfusion
- *steroids*
- *insulin*: maintainance of a blood glucose of around 8 mmol/l improves outcome
- *activated protein C*: this is given to patients at high risk of death secondary to sepsis with shock, multi-organ failure (MOF) or ARDS, where there is no absolute contraindication relating to bleeding, and where there is optimum intensive care support[3]
- *haemofiltration*: to remove inflammatory mediators.

---

3 Activated protein C mediates the clotting cascade which is closely linked to inflammatory pathways. NICE (2004) Drotrecogin alfa (activated) for severe sepsis. It therefore has an anti-inflammatory effect. *NICE Technology Appraisal Guidance* **84.**

The critically ill patient

Referring to ITU/HDU

Refer to ITU/HDU for a higher level of monitoring, when circulatory/respiratory support is required, or if more than one organ system is failing. The patient's condition should be at least partially reversible. Referrals are often required to be consultant-to-consultant. Ensure that all appropriate information is available (including recent blood results and arterial blood gas readings).

Cardiac support

The aim with all critically ill patients is to maximise cardiac function and oxygen delivery to tissues. This will depend on Hb, perfusion pressure and also ventilation and gas exchange. The ability of tissue to utilise the oxygen supplied can be summarised by the oxygen dissociation diagram shown in Figure 3.1, e.g. correcting an acidosis will improve dissociation of O_2 thus improving tissue oxygenation.

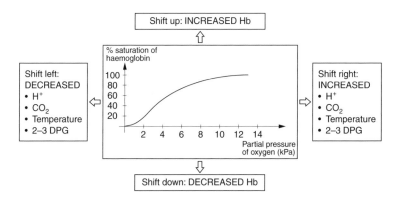

Figure 3.1   Oxygen dissociation curve.

In the critical care setting, invasive monitoring measures such as arterial lines, CVP, and pulmonary artery catheters are used to maximise cardiac efficiency (this will depend on preload, contractility and afterload).

Arterial lines

These provide a beat-to-beat indication of blood pressure allowing early recognition of changes in an unstable patient. They also enable easy access for blood sampling without the need for regular venepuncture. Arterial lines are commonly placed in the radial artery, but if this is not possible, the brachial or dorsalis pedis artery can be used.

Central venous pressure (CVP)

CVP is used as a marker of intravascular volume. It is measured via a central line, placed either in the internal jugular or subclavian veins. The tip of the catheter lies in the superior vena cava just above the opening to the right atrium (look for the tip opposite the hilum or check CXR after placement).

The CVP line therefore provides information regarding right heart filling or 'preload'. Femoral lines can also be used, and pressure measurements here will correlate with central pressure (unless intra-abdominal pressure is increased).

Avoid using the term 'normal CVP' because this only applies to a well patient (where CVP is 0–10 cmH$_2$O). In an unwell patient, vasoconstriction or dilatation can make absolute values difficult to interpret. The trend in CVP is more important than the actual value. The response to a fluid challenge, for example 250 ml colloid, should be assessed if there are concerns that the patient is not adequately filled. The aim is to achieve a sustained rise in CVP following the challenge. This indicates adequate filling has been achieved and therefore, according to Starling's law of the heart,[4] contractility will be maximised. An artificially high CVP may be seen if a shocked patient is rapidly filled due to increased volumes in a vasoconstricted system (see Figure 3.2).

Right-sided pressure does not always reflect left-sided pressure, particularly in critically ill patients, so CVP may not provide a reliable measure of left ventricular preload (which is the main determinant of cardiac output). This is where pulmonary artery catheters may be useful.

Pulmonary artery catheters

Pulmonary artery (PA) catheters (otherwise known as Swan–Ganz catheters) are used to measure cardiac output, ensure optimal fluid resuscitation and guide the use of vasoactive drugs. They are inserted in the same manner as CVP lines, but have a balloon allowing them to float through the right side of the heart to 'wedge' the tip in a distal pulmonary artery. From here there is a continuous column of blood to the left side of the heart, and it can therefore be used as a guide to left heart filling pressure, SVR (systemic vascular resistance) and cardiac output. PA catheters can also be used to measure mixed venous oxygen content, which gives an indication of oxygen delivery and uptake.

---

4 Cardiac output = heart rate × stroke volume. Stroke volume is determined by preload (venous return to the heart), contractility (governed by Starling's law and therefore also dependent on venous return) and after load (peripheral vascular resistance).

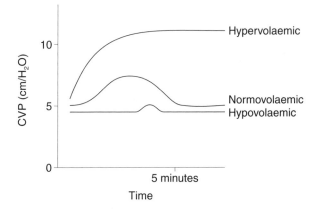

Figure 3.2   Change in CVP as a result of fluid bolus.

Oesophageal Doppler

Cardiac output can also be measured using oesophageal Doppler. A probe is placed in the mid-oesophagus which measures the velocity of blood in the descending aorta. This method is poorly tolerated in awake patients.

Inotropes

Different inotropic agents are used in particular circumstances. Any inotrope may act on several receptors so idiosyncratic responses can occur.

- *Noradrenaline* mainly acts on α_1 receptors causing vasoconstriction and is therefore used in sepsis to counter vasodilation
- *Adrenaline* at low doses acts on β_1 (drives the heart) and β_2 (causes vasodilation) receptors, and so is used for pump failure, but at higher doses will also act on α_1 receptors (causing vasoconstriction)
- *Dobutamine* acts on β_1 and β_2 receptors as adrenaline (however the β_2 effect may predominate resulting in circulatory collapse)
- *Dopamine* acts on β_1, β_2 and dopamine $(DA)_1$ receptors. Classically low dose = 'renal', moderate dose = 'cardiac', and high dose = 'cardiac plus vasoconstriction'. However this is a very simplified scheme. The 'renal' effect of low dose may simply be due to improved general perfusion with increased blood pressure
- *Dopexamine* acts on DA_1 and β_2 receptors.

Respiratory support

Respiratory failure occurs where there is inadequate exchange of O_2 or CO_2 to meet metabolic demands, and is classified as:

- *type 1*: impaired oxygen transfer, hypoxia with low CO_2
- *type 2*: inadequate ventilation, with high CO_2.

In any patient, if hypoxia does not improve with oxygen therapy or the patient is tiring with an increasing PCO_2, further respiratory support may be necessary. There are many methods of support. In a spontaneously breathing patient, continuous positive airways pressure (CPAP) can be used. This provides positive end-expiratory pressure (PEEP), thus preventing alveolar collapse, increasing the working lung volume and reducing the work of breathing. CPAP, however, can result in a fall in cardiac preload due to an increase in mean thoracic pressure. This may be of benefit to patients with cardiac failure, but can cause cardio-vascular collapse in the hypovolaemic patient. Non-invasive positive pressure ventilation (NIPPV) is an alternative and can be delivered via a face mask.

Intubation and ventilation may be required if:

- the patient is tiring with a rising PCO_2
- the patient is unable to maintain their own airway (GCS < 8)
- non-invasive ventilation is contraindicated (e.g. facial trauma), poorly tolerated or fails
- there is a need for suctioning of secretions.

However intubation and ventilation can:

- decrease venous return because of increased intrathoracic pressure
- cause gastric dilatation
- lead to atrophy of respiratory muscles
- cause barotrauma
- result in development of a pneumothorax/surgical emphysema.

A tracheostomy may be necessary to aid weaning or if the duration of ventilation is likely to be prolonged.

Adult respiratory distress syndrome (ARDS)

ARDS occurs in:

- sepsis
- massive blood transfusion
- fat embolism
- trauma
- aspiration
- pneumonia
- pancreatitis
- burns.

There is transudation of fluid in the lungs, thickening of alveolar capillaries and ventilation/perfusion mismatch. A normal pulmonary artery wedge pressure (less than 18 mmHg) distinguishes ARDS from cardiogenic pulmonary oedema.

Renal failure

The causes of renal failure can be classified as:

- *pre-renal*: hypovolaemia, under-perfusion, e.g. in sepsis, renal artery pathology
- *renal*: glomerulonephritis, myoglobin damage secondary to rhabdomyolysis, drugs, e.g. non-steroidal anti-inflammatory drugs (NSAIDs)
- *post-renal*: obstruction secondary to stone, blood clot, urinary retention.

Renal failure may result in:

- *uraemia*: complications include encephalopathy, pericardial effusion
- *fluid overload*
- *electrolyte imbalance* (high potassium).

Treatment of acute renal failure involves:

- *correction of electrolyte disturbances*
- *correction of hypovolaemia*
- *cessation of nephrotoxic drugs*
- *treatment of the underlying cause.*

Renal replacement therapy

Indications for renal replacement therapy in renal failure are:

- *metabolic acidosis, pH < 7.2*
- $K^+ > 6.0\ mmol/l$

- *fluid overload*
- *complications of uraemia.*

Both haemofiltration and haemodialysis can be performed via a dual-lumen central line. In haemofiltration, blood is driven through a semi-permeable membrane. Haemofiltration is better tolerated in patients with cardiovascular disease. Haemodialysis involves the passage of blood over a semi-permeable membrane, allowing equilibrium to occur with dialysis fluid on the other side. Haemodialysis allows quicker correction of acidosis.

Nutrition

In general when oral intake is likely to be absent for more than 5 days the patient will require additional nutritional support.

Enteral feeding[5]

Enteral feeding can be achieved via a nasogastric (NG) tube, nasojejunal tube, percutaneous endoscopic gastrostomy (PEG), or jejunostomy. It can be used in the unconscious patient (e.g. head injury/ventilated patients), those with swallowing disorders, partial intestinal failure (post-operative ileus) and uncomplicated pancreatitis.

Advantages

- Translocation of gut bacteria and villous atrophy is thought to contribute to the development of SIRS in critically ill patients. Early enteral feeding may reduce bacterial translocation and protect gut mucosa, and after major GI surgery has been shown to reduce the incidence of infection (this effect is enhanced by addition of glutamine to feed) and hospital stay[6]
- It is cheaper and easier to manage than parenteral feeding with fewer complications.

Disadvantages

- There is an increased risk of aspiration if there is gastric accumulation. Feeding rate should be reduced if the gastric residue is greater than 200 ml. A prokinetic agent (e.g. metoclopramide) may help
- Enteral feeding commonly causes GI symptoms: nausea (10–20%), abdominal bloating; diarrhoea (30–60%).

---

5   Stroud M, Duncan H and Nightingale J (2003) Guidelines for enteral feeding in adult hospital patients. *Gut* **52** (Suppl 7): vii1–vii12 [Guidelines commissioned by British Society of Gastroenterology].

6   Lewis SJ, Egger M, Sylvester PA and Thomas S (2001) Early enteral feeding versus 'nil by mouth' after gastrointestinal surgery: a systematic review and meta-analysis of controlled trial. *BMJ* **323**: 773–6.

Parenteral feeding (TPN)

Parenteral nutrition is given via a peripheral long line (PICC) or central line. It is given for example in post-operative patients when there is a prolonged ileus, GI fistulae and short bowel syndrome.

Disadvantages

- There is little benefit if used for <7 days
- Venous access is required
- Fatty infiltration of the liver with hepatic impairment can occur. This can progress to fulminant hepatic failure with continued feeding
- Overfeeding. This can increase the risk of sepsis. Excess CO_2 production leads to metabolic acidosis with subsequent increase in respiratory work.

Check daily U&Es and glucose, and weekly LFTs, Ca^{2+}, phosphate and Mg^{2+}.

Stress ulcer prophylaxis should be given to critically ill patients until full enteral nutrition is established. The relative efficacy of H_2 receptor blockers versus proton pump inhibitors (PPIs) has not been evaluated.

Death and organ donation

In order to certify a patient you should document the following:

- absent respiratory effort for 3 min
- absent pulse and heart sounds for 1 min
- fixed dilated pupils.

A hypothermic patient cannot be certified dead until warmed to at least 35°C.

Death certificate

A death certificate can be issued immediately if you feel happy about the cause of death, have seen the patient alive within the last 14 days, and there is no reason to refer to the coroner. If in doubt speak to a senior colleague. Always remember to let the GP know.

Informing the coroner

Inform the coroner in any of the following circumstances:

- the patient died within 24 h of arriving in hospital
- death is caused by a road traffic accident (RTA), industrial disease, violence, suicide, poisoning, neglect or abortion
- surgical procedure within 30 days
- cause of death is unknown
- cause of death is due to a hospital intervention
- death occurred during legal custody or while sectioned under the Mental Health Act
- if there is any claim for negligence against medical or nursing staff
- death due to employment.

The coroner may be happy for the death certificate to be issued, request a post-mortem examination[7] or an inquest.

Brainstem death

Brainstem death is cessation of brain function despite the artificial maintenance of cardiac, respiratory and other organ function.

---

7   Post-mortems requested by the coroner are mandatory by law. These are distinct from hospital post-mortems which may be requested by your consultant. You will need to liaise with the family and the pathologist.

There are strict guidelines governing the diagnosis of brainstem death:

- the patient must be assessed by two doctors. Each must have been registered for at least 5 years and be a registrar or a consultant
- the patient must be unresponsive on a ventilator
- the cause of coma must be known and be irreversible, i.e. excluding drug suppression of CNS, recent shock/hypotension, hypothermia (core temperature must be >35°C)
- check there is no respiratory effort when $PCO_2 > 6.70$ kPa (the 'apnoea' test: disconnect the ventilator with O_2 only via the endotracheal tube)
- check the absence of reflexes: pupillary, corneal, gag, vestibulocochlear (no eye movement after 20 ml iced water to each external auditory meatus with clear access to the tympanic membrane)
- check there are no motor responses to cranial nerve stimulation.

Organ donation

For a patient to be considered for organ donation there needs to be a diagnosis of brainstem death along with an intact circulation. The cause of death in such cases is usually trauma, intracerebral bleed, or primary brain tumour (proven on histology). Patients are excluded from donation if there is a neoplasm other than a primary brain tumour, HIV, hepatitis B/C, generalised infection, or diabetes.

Once a donor has been identified, brainstem death must be confirmed. Contact the transplant co-ordinating team who will then help in discussion with the patient's family, check HIV, hepatitis B/C, blood group (heart, lung and liver transplants are matched this way) and tissue typing (only necessary for renal transplants).

Chapter 4
Trauma

Trauma[1]

ABC approach to the trauma patient (primary survey)

A: Airway and cervical spine control

On approaching the patient immobilise the neck manually until secured while assessing the airway.

Assess the airway:

- if the patient can speak to you the airway is patent. If unable to speak inspect for foreign body/facial trauma
- try chin lift/jaw thrust.

If these measures are inadequate consider an *oral/nasal airway:*

- oropharangeal or Guedel airway (sized from corner of mouth to the tragus)
- nasal airway (do not use in a head injury/basal skull fracture. Sized according to little finger).

If these measures are inadequate a *definitive airway* is required. A definitive airway is defined as a cuffed tube placed in the trachea, with the cuff inflated connected to an oxygen supply and secured with tape.

A *surgical airway* is indicated if the trachea cannot be intubated, e.g. due to oedema, oropharyngeal bleeding or severe maxillofacial injury. This can be achieved either temporarily by jet insufflation,[2] or by surgical cricothyroidotomy.[3]

Once the airway is established administer oxygen at 15 l/min, and ensure adequate oxygenation during attempts at intubation.

Immobilise the head and neck (use a correctly sized collar, 'sandbags' and two lengths of tape to immobilise the cervical spine).[4]

B: Breathing and ventilation

- *Expose the chest*

---

1 *See* American College of Surgeons (1997) *Advanced Trauma Life Support (ATLS) Guidelines* (6e). American College of Surgeons, Chicago.
2 A 12–14G cannula is inserted through the cricothyroid membrane and attached to 15 l O_2. A Y connector is covered for 1 s and released for 4 s to allow expiration. CO_2 inevitably accumulates, and so this method can only be used for 30–45 min.
3 Surgical cricothyroidotomy is performed via a small incision through the cricothyroid membrane and insertion of a small E-T tube or tracheostomy tube.
4 The cervical spine can only be 'cleared' if the patient is fully conscious, with no head injury, no neck pain, no distracting injury, no abnormal neurology and no history of drugs/alcohol.

- Check the *trachea is central*
- Watch chest for *asymmetrical or paradoxical movement*[5]
- Palpate for *tenderness*
- Check *expansion*
- *Percuss* and *auscultate.*

Tension pneumothorax

Features are:

- chest pain
- shortness of breath (SOB)
- tachycardia
- hypotension
- trachea deviated away from the affected side
- reduced or absent chest movement on the affected side
- percussion is hyper-resonant
- breath sounds are reduced.

Immediate *needle thoracocentesis* must be performed.[6]

Open pneumothorax

If there is an open injury to the chest with a diameter of more than two-thirds the diameter of the trachea, then air will preferentially enter the pleural cavity via the defect. Initial management involves taping an occlusive dressing over the wound on three sides to act as a flutter valve. A chest drain should be inserted distant from the wound.[7]

Haemothorax

Haemothorax is accumulation of blood in the pleural cavity. Features are as for tension pneumothorax except percussion is dull rather than resonant. There may

---

5   A flail segment exists when two or more adjacent ribs fracture in two or more places, creating a segment of chest wall that moves paradoxically with respiration. This impairs ventilation and is often associated with a significant underlying pulmonary contusion.
6   Insert a large-bore cannula into the 2nd intercostal space in the midclavicular line of the affected side. This converts a tension pneumothorax into a simple pneumothorax for which a chest drain should subsequently be inserted.
7   Normally inserted into the 5th intercostal space in the anterior axillary line. Use at least size 32 Fr in trauma.

be features of hypovolaemic shock. A chest drain should be inserted. If there is more than 1.5 l of blood loss immediately or >200 ml/h for 2–4 h, thoracotomy is indicated (contact cardiothoracic surgeons).

Pulmonary contusion

This is bruising to the lung. Pulmonary contusion may lead to progressive respiratory failure. Ensure adequate pain control and consider intubation and ventilation early if the patient's clinical condition deteriorates.

C: Circulation and haemorrhage control

- *Check pulse* and *blood pressure*
- *Insert two large venous cannulae* and *send bloods*: FBC, U&Es, LFTs, glucose, clotting, cross-match blood
- *Consider potential sites of significant blood loss* (chest, abdomen, pelvis, long bones, retroperitoneum).

Remember that neck veins may not be an accurate guide to fluid-filling status in trauma. They may be distended in tension pneumothorax/tamponade despite hypovolaemia.

Fluid resuscitation and control of haemorrhage

Give 2 litres of warmed Hartmann's. As the patient is fluid resuscitated the increasing blood pressure may result in further haemorrhage/clot displacement (this is the theory behind 'low volume pre-hospital resuscitation').[8]
   Remember the following:

- visible external haemorrhage should be controlled by direct pressure
- tourniquets should never be used.

Examine the abdomen and pelvis:

- blunt abdominal injury may result in rupture of hollow organs/diaphragm
- deceleration injuries include lacerations of the liver and spleen
- a pelvic fracture implies a high-force injury,[9] and is often associated with visceral/retroperitoneal injury. Disruption of presacral or pelvic vessels can account for significant concealed blood loss.

---

8 In pre-hospital care i.v. fluids should not be administered if the radial pulse is palpable; 250 ml bolus crystalloid if absent. *See* NICE (2004) Prehospital Initiation of Fluid Replacement Therapy in Trauma. *NICE Technology Appraisal Guidance* TA074.

Cardiac tamponade

The pericardium fills with blood and restricts cardiac output. Cardiac tamponade can be easily confused clinically with tension pneumothorax (as it causes respiratory distress, tachycardia, hypotension and distended neck veins). The classical picture of Beck's triad (hypotension, dilated neck veins and muffled heart sounds) is less useful in trauma. Tamponade may be quickly diagnosed using USS or echocardiogram (ECHO), if immediately available. However it may be necessary to proceed directly to pericardiocentesis.[10]

Cardiac contusion

This is caused by blunt cardiac injury and often associated with rib or sternal fractures and cardiac tamponade. There may be ECG changes and dysrhythmias.

Aortic disruption

There should be a high index of suspicion of aortic injury following a fall or high-speed deceleration injury.

Look for the following CXR signs:

- widened mediastinum
- haemothorax
- 1st/2nd rib or scapula fracture
- obliteration of the aortic knob
- tracheal deviation to the right
- presence of a pleural cap
- elevation of the right and depression of the left main bronchus
- deviation of the oesophagus to the right.

An aortic rupture that survives to hospital is usually an incomplete contained rupture. The cardiothoracic team should be involved immediately.

---

9 Assessment of the pelvis for instability should only be performed once, as this may displace any blood clots that have formed. Temporary stabilisation, using a sheet of antishock garment, can afford temporary control of blood loss prior to surgical stabilisation.

10 Insertion of a spinal needle attached to a syringe 1–2 cm below the xiphisternum at 45° aimed towards the tip of the scapula. The syringe should be aspirated during insertion. Watch the cardiac monitor as arrhythmias may occur if the needle touches the myocardium.

D: Disability

Neurological status can be assessed quickly using AVPU:

A = Alert
V = responds to Voice
P = responds to Pain
U = Unresponsive to all stimuli.

A more quantifiable method of assessing neurological status is the GCS (Glasgow Coma Scale). *See* page 74.

E: Exposure and environmental control

Fully *expose the patient*: take measures to *prevent hypothermia* (warm fluids, cover with blanket/warming sheet, use heat lamps).

Adjuncts to the primary survey

- *X-rays* should be taken in the following order:
  1 *chest*
  2 *pelvis*
  3 *lateral C-spine*
- *Pulse oximetry*
- *ECG monitoring*
- Insert a *urinary catheter* (contraindicated if there is evidence of urethral trauma)
- A *NGT* may be inserted to reduce the risk of aspiration.

Secondary survey

Once the patient is stable a full top-to-toe examination should be performed:

- *a full neurological examination*
- *check the scalp* for lacerations, contusions, and evidence of underlying skull fracture (depression/boggy swelling)
- *examine the face and eyes* (bruising + oedema may lead to closing of the eyes making later examination difficult)
- *check the pupils, eye movements, acuity, corneal abrasions, and remove contact lenses*
- *examine for evidence of bruising, tenderness and diminished breath signs over the chest wall*

- *examine the abdomen*, and look for tenderness, bruising and distension
- *examine the pelvis, perineum and genitalia*
- a *log roll* should be performed to allow full examination of the *spine* and a *rectal examination*
- examine the *peripheral limbs* for pulses, swelling, bruising, deformity and tenderness.

The agitated patient

Causes of agitation in a trauma patient include hypoxia, hypovolaemia, hypoglycaemia, head injury (cerebral oedema), pain, intoxication, full bladder, tight dressings. The patient may have taken alcohol/drugs, but always look for other causes first.

Trauma and pregnancy

Physiological changes in pregnancy alter some aspects of trauma management:

- there is already an increased pulse and reduced blood pressure (BP) (in the 2nd trimester)
- plasma volume is increased by up to 20% with an increased cardiac output, so a greater volume will have to be lost before signs of shock become evident
- a small degree of hyperventilation may be normal.

In all cases the mother should be treated first:

- if the mother is shocked, blood may be diverted away from the foetus
- the mother should be treated where possible in the left lateral position, or with the pelvis tilted to prevent foetal compression of the inferior vena cava (IVC)
- X-rays should still be taken in the emergency setting
- anti-D should be given to Rhesus-negative mothers following trauma.

Abdominal trauma

Abdominal trauma may be either:

- *blunt*: e.g. road traffic accidents
- *penetrating*: e.g. stab wounds, gunshot injuries.

Blunt trauma

Mechanism of injury

- Compression/crushing (solid or distended organ, e.g. liver, full bladder)
- Shearing
- Deceleration (e.g. liver and spleen at site of supporting ligaments).

Most frequent injuries

- Spleen
- Liver
- Retroperitoneal haematoma.

Penetrating trauma

Mechanism of injury

- Direct
- Indirect (e.g. cavitation from high-velocity bullet).

Most frequent injuries

- Liver
- Small bowel
- Colon
- Diaphragm
- Abdominal vascular structures.

History and examination

A significant abdominal injury is likely if there is:

- a relevant mechanism of injury
- abdominal pain that may be referred to the shoulder

- unexplained hypotension
- a penetrating wound to the lower chest, abdomen or perineum/gluteal region
- bruising of the abdominal wall/flanks
- a seatbelt sign[11]
- peritonism
- absent bowel sounds (unreliable)
- blood on digital rectal examination (DRE)
- related injury (e.g. chest or pelvis).

Management

Follow ABC and resuscitate the patient. A basic algorithm for managing abdominal trauma is shown in Figure 4.1.

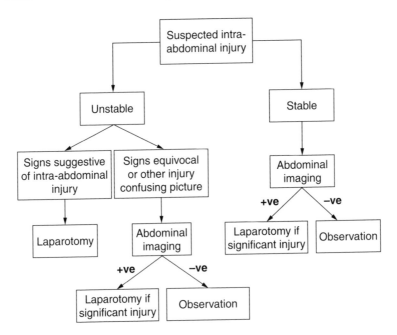

Figure 4.1 Basic algorithm for managing abdominal trauma.

---

11 Linear ecchymosis in the line of a restraining seatbelt. Suggests significant deceleration force.

The stable patient

Blunt injury

- Look for free air under the diaphragm on erect CXR
- Consider abdominal imaging (CT or USS of the abdomen)[12]
- If a significant injury is demonstrated, proceed to laparotomy
- If the injury is not significant, admit for observation and serial clinical examinations
- Consider contrast study if you suspect injury to retroperitoneal bowel (e.g. duodenum) not demonstrated on CT.

Penetrating injury

- Look for free air under the diaphragm on erect CXR
- Explore the wound (under LA or GA)
- Patients with wounds on the back or flank that are not obviously superficial should be admitted for serial clinical examinations or evaluated with contrast enhanced CT
- If the wound has entered the peritoneal cavity consider laparotomy.[13]

The unstable patient

If an abdominal injury is the most likely cause, proceed to laparotomy without delay.

Indications for laparotomy

- Blunt trauma with recurrent hypotension despite adequate resuscitation
- Blunt trauma with significant injury on CT scan (or contrast study)
- Penetrating trauma with hypotension
- Bleeding from the stomach, rectum or genitourinary tract following penetrating injury
- Early or subsequent peritonitis
- Evisceration

---

12 CT is more sensitive than USS with regard to specific organ injuries. Ultrasonography has clear advantages over diagnostic peritoneal lavage as an initial investigation in blunt abdominal trauma. *See* Jansen JO and Logie JRC (2005) Diagnostic peritoneal lavage – an obituary. *Br J Surg* **92**: 517–18.
13 Not all patients with penetrating wounds that enter the peritoneal cavity will necessarily require a laparotomy. An alternative approach is to admit for serial clinical examinations with surgery reserved for those who deteriorate.

- Gunshot wounds traversing the peritoneal cavity/retroperitoneum
- Radiological evidence of perforated viscus or ruptured diaphragm.

Additional features of specific organ injury

Hepatic injuries

- Mechanism: e.g. penetrating injury to right lower chest/right upper quadrant/right flank *or* deceleration injury
- Lower right rib fracture(s) +/– raised right hemidiaphragm on CXR.

Splenic injuries

- Increased risk with splenomegaly
- Mechanism: e.g. direct blow to lower left chest *or* deceleration injury
- Lower left rib fracture/s, displaced gastric bubble, raised left hemidiaphragm, and pleural effusion on CXR
- Loss of left psoas shadow, medially displaced left kidney on AXR.

Duodenum and pancreas[14]

- Mechanism: e.g. direct blow to epigastrium *or* deceleration injury (duodenum)
- Haematemesis/blood aspirated via NG tube (duodenum)
- Air outlining retroperitoneal structures on AXR (duodenum)
- Elevation of the left hemidiaphragm, pleural effusion on CXR (pancreas)
- Lower thoracic spine injury (pancreas).

Other bowel injuries

- Mechanism: e.g. penetrating injury *or* deceleration injury
- Blood aspirated via NG tube (stomach), or rectal bleeding
- Free air on CXR or AXR
- Lumbar distraction fracture (Chance fracture, small bowel).

Diaphragm

- Mechanism: e.g. compression injury (left hemidiaphragm most commonly affected) *or* penetrating injury

---

14 Serum amylase is not a reliable marker of pancreatic injury.

- Elevation, irregularity or obliteration of part or all of the diaphragm, mass *or* abnormal gas shadow above the diaphragm (herniation of abdominal contents into chest), pleural effusion, contralateral mediastinal shift, widening of cardiac shadow (herniation into pericardial sac) and lower rib fractures on CXR.

Urological trauma

Injuries to the genitourinary tract occur in approximately 10% of major trauma.

Renal injuries

- The majority are of a minor nature
- Severe injuries can occur after high-speed injuries (e.g. motorbike), and are usually associated with rib fracture and damage to other neighbouring organs.

Signs

- *Haematuria*[15] (90%)
- *Flank ecchymosis.*

Specific investigations

- AXR may show absence of psoas shadow, enlarged kidney, fracture of 10th/11th/12th ribs or L1–3 transverse processes, and scoliosis to the affected side
- CT is the investigation of choice. This should be performed after blunt injury in patients with:
  - macroscopic haematuria
  - hypotension and microscopic haematuria
  - microscopic haematuria and the presence of significant injury to other organs
- An *IVU* is an alternative in haemodynamically stable patients, but provides less information than a CT scan.

Classification of renal injuries

- *Type I*: minor contusion
- *Type II*: minor parenchymal laceration; no involvement of collecting system
- *Type III*: major laceration; collecting system involved
- *Type IV*: renal pedicle injury.

---

15 Major renal injuries in adults invariably present with haematuria and shock.

Management

The majority of renal trauma are type I and II injuries, and can usually be managed conservatively.

Indications for surgery

Surgery may be indicated if there is major injury (type III or IV). Before laparotomy it is preferable to ensure adequate function of the contralateral kidney by CT, in case nephrectomy is necessary.

Absolute indications for renal exploration are:

- haemorrhage occurring from a renal injury
- avulsion of the renal pedicle
- expanding retroperitoneal haematoma.

Exploration *may* be required if there is:

- a large laceration to the renal pelvis
- co-existing organ injury
- persistent urinary leakage which cannot be managed non-operatively
- renal artery thrombosis
- renal vascular injuries.

Ureteric injury

- Usually iatrogenic but can occur after penetrating injuries
- Often initially identified at laparotomy
- Most injuries can be repaired with primary anastomosis over a ureteric stent. Rarely a urinary diversion procedure is required.

Bladder injuries

In blunt trauma, bladder injury is usually associated with pelvic fracture.[16]

Symptoms and signs

- *Abdominal pain*
- *Haematuria*
- *Inability to urinate.*

---

16 10% of patients with a pelvic fracture will have associated bladder or urethral injury.

Specific investigations

- *Anterior–posterior (A–P) pelvic X-ray*
- *IVU* followed by retrograde cystogram/CT *cystography.*

Management

- *Extraperitoneal rupture* can often be *managed conservatively* with bladder drainage
- *Intraperitoneal rupture* (most common in trauma) usually *requires exploration and repair.*

Urethral injuries

These can be either *anterior* (bulbar and penile urethra) or *posterior* (prostatic and membranous urethra), and invariably occur in males (the male urethra is far longer than in the female). Posterior injuries are usually associated with pelvic fracture.

Symptoms and signs

- *Blood at the urethral meatus*
- *High-riding prostate* on DRE
- Evidence of *perineal urinoma or haematoma.*

Specific investigations

- *Retrograde urethrogram*
- *USS* may be useful to look for a pelvic haematoma.

Management

- *Anterior injuries* if minor can be initially managed with *urethral catheterisation* performed by an experienced urologist. Severe injuries may require exploration
- *Posterior injuries* should be treated with *urinary diversion* (suprapubic catheter) in the first instance. *Urethroscopy* +/– repair may be necessary later.

Vascular trauma

This may be due to *penetrating* (gunshot/stabbing) or *blunt* injury (in association with fractures or crush injury).

Extremity injuries

Vascular extremity injuries are often associated with orthopaedic injuries, most commonly dislocation of the knee and supracondylar/proximal tibial fracture.

Symptoms and signs

- *Bruit*
- *Haemorrhage*
- *Ischaemia of the limb* (+/– presence of a peripheral pulse[17]).

Management

- *Resuscitate and control haemorrhage* with direct pressure
- *Immediate surgery*[18] *if there is a clear vascular injury*
- *Consider pre-operative or on-table angiography* to confirm the presence and extent of the injury.

Neck vascular injuries

These are usually associated with penetrating injuries. Carotid artery injuries account for about 10% of vascular injuries. Establish a safe airway and control haemorrhage by compression if possible. Continuing haemorrhage merits early exploration with an on-table angiogram if necessary.

---

17 The presence of a distal pulse does not rule out a peripheral vascular injury.
18 Vascular repair may involve simple end-to-end suturing, vein patch or interposition graft using vein or PTFE. Fasciotomy may be necessary either for prevention or treatment of compartment syndrome.

Spinal trauma

Suspect a spinal cord injury if there has been a fall or high-speed injury. Up to 20% of spinal cord injuries occur at more than one level. With a suspected spinal injury keep the patient immobilised, and maintain good BP/oxygenation.

The injury may be *complete* or *incomplete*.

A *complete* spinal injury may result in *neurogenic shock*. Features include:

- bradycardia
- hypotension
- diaphragmatic breathing
- priapism.

Incomplete spinal injury (*see* Figure 4.2) may result in:

- *Brown–Séquard syndrome*: this is often due to a penetrating injury and occurs because of hemisection of the cord with loss of ascending and descending spinal cord tracts on that side. There are bilateral signs with ipsilateral paralysis and loss of proprioception, and contralateral loss of pain and temperature sensation
- *central cord syndrome*: usually due to a hyperextension injury in a patient with long-standing cervical spondylosis. This affects decussating fibres of the spinothalamic tract. Medial fibres are affected first, and therefore motor and sensory impairment in the upper extremities is usually greater than in the lower extremities. Characteristically there is 'sacral sparing'
- *anterior cord syndrome*: due to a flexion injury. This results in motor paralysis and loss of pain/temperature sensation. Proprioception is intact.

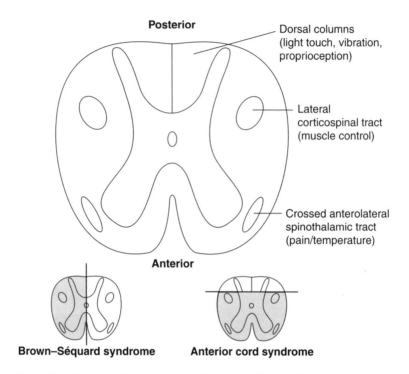

Posterior

Dorsal columns
(light touch, vibration,
proprioception)

Lateral
corticospinal tract
(muscle control)

Crossed anterolateral
spinothalamic tract
(pain/temperature)

Anterior

Brown–Séquard syndrome   **Anterior cord syndrome**

Figure 4.2   Cross-section of the spinal cord, and the site of common lesions.

Assessment of a head injury

Many hospitals use a proforma for the assessment of head injuries.

History

Record the following:

- age
- events that occurred
- loss of consciousness (LOC)
- amnesia (retrograde, antegrade, length)
- presence of headache
- visual disturbance
- nausea and vomiting (how many times)
- seizures
- use of aspirin/anticoagulants (bleeding tendency)
- use of alcohol and drugs.

Examination

- As for trauma: *ABC, with C spine protection* (5% of head injuries have an associated neck injury)
- Assess *Glasgow Coma Scale* (GCS) – *see* Table 4.1
- *Boggy swelling* of the scalp may suggest an underlying *skull fracture*
- Also look for signs of a *basal skull fracture*.[19]

---

19 Signs include periorbital haematomas (Panda eyes), Battle's sign (bruising behind ears), CSF rhinorrhoea or ottorhoea, haemotympanum (bleeding behind the tympanic membrane).

Table 4.1   The Glasgow Coma Scale

Eye opening	Verbal response	Motor response
4 = Spontaneous	5 = Normal conversation	6 = Normal
3 = To voice	4 = Disoriented conversation	5 = Localises to pain
2 = To pain	3 = Words, but not coherent	4 = Withdraws to pain
1 = None	2 = No words. Only sounds	3 = Decorticate posture
	1 = None	2 = Decerebrate
		1 = None

Score = eye opening + verbal response + motor response

Minimum score is 3 and maximum score 15. The best response should be recorded.

Mild head injury GCS 13–15; **Moderate head injury** GCS 9–12; **Severe head injury** GCS < 8.[20]

Investigations

- *Skull X-ray*[21]: a skull fracture is associated with a significant risk of intracranial haematoma, but CT is now the investigation of choice for head injuries
- *CT head*: CT scan can be used to detect intracranial haematoma, brain swelling or shift, intracranial air/fracture.

Indications for CT

- *Significant mechanism of injury* (fall from height, ejection from vehicle)
- *Reduced level of consciousness* (GCS < 13 at any point after injury or 13/14 more than 2 h after injury)
- *Focal neurological signs*
- *Seizures*
- *Suspected open or depressed skull fracture*
- *Signs of basal skull fracture*

---

20 GCS < 8 is generally accepted as 'coma'. The patient will be unable to protect their own airway and will therefore require intubation.

21 NICE guidelines recommend CT scanning as the preferred investigation. However a skull X-ray may be helpful when CT facilities are not available, or if there is concern regarding the mechanism of injury (e.g. non-accidental injury in children). *See* www.nice.org.uk: *Head Injury: triage, assessment, investigation and early management of head injury in infants, children and adults.* Guideline CG4. London: NICE.

- *Greater than 30 min of retrograde amnesia*
- *More than one episode of vomiting*
- *Predisposition to bleeding* (e.g. patient anticoagulated).

Intracranial haematoma

The risk of intracranial bleeding is shown in Table 4.2.

Table 4.2   Risk of intracranial bleeding

Neurological status	Fracture	Risk
GCS 15	No	<1:1000
GCS 15	Yes	1:30
Confused	No	1:100
Confused	Yes	1:5
Coma	Yes	1:4

Expansion of an intracranial haematoma results in increased intracranial pressure (ICP). This can lead to herniation of the brain, e.g. in a unilateral expanding haematoma the medial temporal lobe is displaced through the tentorial hiatus leading to a reduced consciousness level, dilated ipsilateral pupil (IIIrd nerve compression), and later ptosis with deviation of the eye (down and out).

With a diffuse rise in intracranial pressure, herniation of the cerebellar tonsils occurs causing brainstem compression (coning). This results in dysfunction of cardiorespiratory control with subsequent brainstem death. Cushing's reflex (increase in blood pressure and reduced pulse rate) associated with abnormal respiration and posturing are late responses and shortly precede coning.

Types of haematoma

- *Subdural haematoma*: blood accumulates between the dura and arachnoid mater, forming a crescent-shaped collection which spreads around this potential space. Subdural haematoma is more common than extradural and more severe, with a 35–45% mortality. Haemorrhage commonly arises from a bridging vein between the cortex and venous sinuses. Underlying brain injury and swelling may lead to a midline shift out of proportion to the size of the haematoma itself, and is associated with a worse prognosis.
- *Extradural haematoma*: blood accumulates in the extradural space and therefore has a lentiform appearance on CT. A classic 'lucid interval' is described where the patient appears to improve shortly before death. Extradural haemorrhage often results from damage to the meningeal vessels (especially the middle meningeal artery) over the temporal fossa. If evacuated,

the prognosis is better than with a subdural haematoma as there is usually less associated direct injury to the brain itself.

- *Brain contusion*: haematoma can occur within the substance of the brain itself, e.g. contracoup injury, commonly of the frontal lobe against the anterior cranial fossa or tip of the temporal lobe against the sphenoid wing.

Diffuse brain injury

Diffuse brain injury occurs due to acceleration/deceleration injury, and varies in severity from mild concussion to diffuse axonal injury.

- *Mild concussion*: to make a diagnosis of mild concussion there must be no reduction in consciousness level, with temporary and mild symptoms only, including confusion, disorientation and retrograde/antegrade amnesia.
- *Classical concussion*: there may be a short period of loss of consciousness, with post-traumatic amnesia, the length of which indicates the severity of injury. A post-concussion syndrome may occur. This includes lethargy, memory problems, dizziness, nausea and depression. Up to one-third of patients with a mild head injury have some symptoms of memory, sleep or sexual disturbance.
- *Diffuse axonal injury*: post-traumatic coma which is not due to haematoma or ischaemia, although it may occur in combination with ischaemic damage.

Management of head injury

The general principles of trauma management apply to any head injury: maintain oxygenation and cerebral perfusion by avoidance of hypoxia and hypotension.

Indications for admission to hospital

A patient should be admitted for observation in the following circumstances:

- *no responsible adult at home, or long distance from hospital*
- *altered consciousness level even if CT is normal*
- *abnormal CT* (discuss with neurosurgeons – *see* page 79)
- when *CT is indicated but delayed*
- suspicion of a *basal skull fracture/CSF leak*
- *anticoagulation* (taking warfarin).

If the patient requires admission, 'neuro obs' should be performed every 30 min until the GCS is 15 for more than 2 h. Then reduce the frequency of obs to hourly for 4 h, and 2-hourly thereafter if there is no deterioration.

'Neuro obs' record

- GCS
- Pupil size and reactivity
- Pulse
- Blood pressure
- Temperature
- Respiratory rate
- O_2 saturations
- Limb movement.

A patient may only be discharged if fully alert and orientated with no indication for CT, or following a normal scan. Ensure that there is a responsible adult at home for the next 48 h and issue *written head injury advice* to return if there is:

- worsening headache not relieved by simple analgesia
- persistent vomiting
- increasing drowsiness or unconsciousness
- fitting
- blurred vision.

Indications for intubation

- *GCS < 8, loss of gag reflex* (unable to protect own airway), or *falling level of consciousness*
- *Seizures*
- *To correct hypoxia* (PaO_2 < 9 kPa on air or < 13 kPa on oxygen) *or hypercapnia* (PaO_2 > 6 kPa). High CO_2 levels result in vasodilation and therefore raised ICP. Previously, patients were hyperventilated to reduce CO_2 levels to below normal, to limit intracranial volume. However, this has been shown to result in vasoconstriction and cerebral ischaemia with a worse prognosis.[22] Current recommendations are to avoid hypercapnia, and not to induce hypocapnia
- *Spontaneous hyperventilation* (with PaO_2 < 3.5 kPa)
- *Respiratory arrhythmias* (e.g. Cheyne–Stokes breathing)
- *Other injury causing airway concern.*

Raised intracranial pressure

Normal intracranial pressure is 0–10 mmHg. A small rise in intracranial volume can be compensated for by CSF displacement without significant increase in ICP. However, beyond a critical volume ICP rises rapidly, resulting in reduced brain perfusion and coning (*see* Figure 4.3).

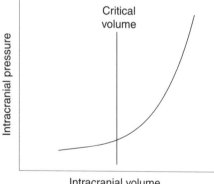

Figure 4.3   Relationship between intracranial volume and intracranial pressure.

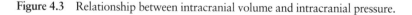

22 Muizelaar JP, Marmarou A, Ward JD *et al.* (1991) Adverse effects of prolonged hyperventilation in patients with severe head injury: a randomised controlled trial. *J Neurosurg* **75**: 731–9.

To minimise the rise in ICP:

- control pain
- prevent coughing (paralyse if intubated/ventilated)
- maintain optimal oxygenation and normal PaO_2.

Prognosis is improved if ICP is kept <20 mmHg and cerebral perfusion pressure >70 mmHg.

Burr holes

The aim of a burr hole is to prevent death by decompressing and partially evacuating a haematoma, e.g. an extradural haematoma due to laceration of the middle meningeal artery.

Burr holes should only be performed by an experienced clinician (because creating a burr hole may itself cause damage), and should never delay transfer to a neurosurgical unit.

Getting neurosurgical assistance

The indications for referral to a neurosurgical centre are:

- coma that persists after the patient has been resuscitated
- unexplained confusion for >4 h regardless of imaging
- significant CT abnormality which may require surgical intervention, e.g. haematoma
- deterioration or progression of signs, e.g. falling GCS, increased confusion
- skull fracture which is depressed or associated with reduced GCS/seizures
- definite or suspected penetrating injury
- CSF leak.

Request neurosurgical advice if in doubt.

When making the referral, the neurosurgeon will need the following information:

- details of the mechanism of injury
- time since injury
- examination findings (cardiorespiratory as well as neurological)
- patient factors (age, anticoagulation, other injuries)
- initial management
- CT results (scans may need to be sent electronically).

During transfer the patient should be accompanied by an anaesthetist. The neurosurgeons may require the patient to be intubated and ventilated prior to transfer. Don't forget to send the notes and films with the patient.

Burns

As the surgeon on call you may be involved in the resuscitation and transfer of burns patients.

Definition

Coagulative destruction of the surface layers of the body.

Incidence

10 000 admissions per year in the UK. Approximately 1000 deaths.[23]

Pathophysiology

Following a burn the necrotic cells and denatured proteins initiate both local and systemic inflammatory responses leading to increased capillary permeability and interstitial fluid/oedema.

Classification

Burns may be classified by:

- *aetiology*: thermal[24] (80–90%), electrical (5–10%), chemical (5–10%)
- *depth*: partial or full-thickness:
  - *partial thickness* burns involve the epidermis and some of the dermis. If only the superficial dermis is involved the skin is red, blistered, blanches with pressure and is very tender. If the majority of the dermis is involved the skin is paler and will be slower to re-epithelialise
  - *full-thickness* burns involve the whole dermis and are dark in appearance. Pin-prick sensation is reduced with deep dermal burns and absent in full-thickness burns
- *percentage body area*: calculate using rule of nines in adults – *see* Figure 4.4.

---

23 Risk of death can be estimated as percentage burn + age (or more accurately using Bull and Fisher tables). *See* Bull JP and Fisher AJ (1954) A study of mortality in a burns unit: a revised estimate. *Ann Surg* **139**: 269–74.
24 The degree of tissue necrosis is proportional to temperature and duration of exposure.

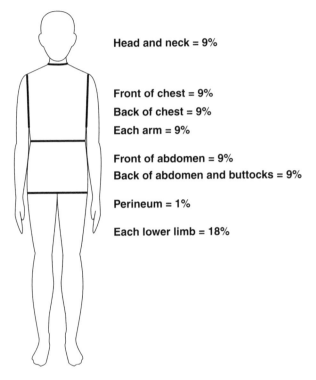

Head and neck = 9%

Front of chest = 9%
Back of chest = 9%
Each arm = 9%

Front of abdomen = 9%
Back of abdomen and buttocks = 9%

Perineum = 1%

Each lower limb = 18%

Figure 4.4   The rule of nines.

Management

Resuscitate as for any trauma patient with particular reference to the following.

- *Airway*: assess risk factors for airway compromise (including burns to nose/mouth, singed nasal hair, hoarse voice, oedema mouth/face, stridor – late sign), and if any of these are present call an anaesthetist
- *Breathing*: assess risk factors for inhalation injury (including significant smoke inhalation, fire in an enclosed space, carbon in sputum, perioral burn, reduced level of consciousness, respiratory distress, carboxyhaemoglobin > 15%). Perform ABGs, a CXR, and consider bronchoscopy. If there is inhalational injury consider nebulised heparin (prevents fibrin plugging), acetylcysteine (mucolytic) and bronchodilators.

- *Circulation*: fluid resuscitation is necessary for >10% burns in children and >15% in adults. Calculate fluid requirements[25] using the Parkland formula (for adults):
  - *4 ml/kg for every 1% burn of normal saline or Hartmann's over 24 h* – the first half should be given over 8 h, and the remainder over the next 16 h. Check electrolytes – these may be deranged. Catheterise the patient and check hourly urine output as a guide to resuscitation. Check 4-hourly Hb and haematocrit. Occasionally a blood transfusion is necessary.

Other treatment considerations

- *Tetanus immunisation*
- *Dressings* to reduce exudate
- *NGT* should be inserted to decompress the stomach as there is a risk of gastric distension, and for enteral feeding when necessary
- Full-thickness circumferential burns require *escharotomy* within 6 h
- Infection: responsible for about half of burn deaths. Risk may be reduced by early wound debridement and closure/grafting. *Topical antimicrobials*, e.g. flamazine, may be used. *Systemic antibiotics* are only required for proven sepsis.

Criteria for transfer to a burns centre

- *Large size dermal or full-thickness burn* (>10% in adults, >5% in children)
- *Children under 5 years*
- *Burns involving face, hands, feet or perineum*
- *Inhalational injury*
- *Chemical and electrical burns*
- *Circumferential burns*
- *Burns in patients with significant co-morbidity or associated injuries* (e.g. fracture).

Complications of burns

- *Infection*
- *Electrolyte disturbances/catabolic state*
- *Respiratory failure* (as a result of inhalation injury or ARDS)

---

25 Fluid requirements will be increased if there is delayed/inadequate initial resuscitation or deep (electrical/petrol) burn, and if there is inhalation injury.

- *DVT/pulmonary embolism* (PE)
- *Rhabdomyolysis*
- *Pancreatitis*
- *Acalculous cholecystitis.*

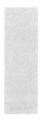

Chapter 5
Hernias

Hernias

Definition

The protrusion of a viscus or part of a viscus, through its containing wall.

Inguinal hernia

The hernial sac emerges *superior* and *medial* to the *pubic tubercle*.

- It is the most common groin hernia in both males and females.
- There is a male to female predominance of approximately 5:1 in infants; 10:1 in adults in the UK.
- It is more common on the right than the left side at all ages (ratio 5:4).
- The incidence of strangulation is estimated to be between 0.3% and 3% per year.[1]
- It is classified as *indirect* or *direct* depending on the relationship of the hernial sac to the inferior epigastric artery.

Indirect inguinal hernia

The hernial sac passes *lateral* to the *inferior epigastric artery* through the deep ring of the inguinal canal:

- it accounts for virtually all groin hernias in infants (incidence approximately 2%)
- it is twice as common as direct hernias in adults (occurs most frequently in younger men)
- it occurs as frequently as femoral hernias in women
- it commonly extends into the scrotum (inguinoscrotal hernia)
- the incidence of strangulation is at least 10 times higher than for a direct inguinal hernia.

Risk factors

Prematurity, twins, low birth weight, ethnicity (higher incidence in patients of African origin).

---

1 Royal College of Surgeons (1993) *Clinical Guidelines for the Management of Groin Hernia in Adults*. Report of a working party convened by the Royal College of Surgeons of England. London: Royal College of Surgeons.

Pathogenesis

Congenital. The sac is the remains of part or all of the processus vaginalis. In infants all inguinal hernias result from intrauterine failure of the processus vaginalis to close. In adults, a patent processus vaginalis opens under the stress of raised intra-abdominal pressure (saccular theory of Russell).

Direct inguinal hernia

The hernial sac passes *medial* to the *inferior epigastric artery* through a defect in the posterior wall of the inguinal canal:

- it occurs most frequently in older males
- it is exceptionally rare in women
- it rarely extends into the scrotum.

Risk factors

Smoking, chronic obstructive pulmonary disease (COPD), aortic aneurysm, connective tissue disease.

Pathogenesis

It is thought to occur because of an acquired weakness in the posterior abdominal wall. The hernial sac passes directly forward through a defect in the posterior wall of the inguinal canal.

Femoral hernia

The hernial sac emerges *through the femoral canal* and therefore passes *inferior and lateral* to the *pubic tubercle*.

- Incidence increases with age (uncommon before 50 years).
- There is a female to male predominance of 2.5:1 in the UK.
- It is more common on the right than the left side at all ages (ratio 5:4).
- The sac may emerge from the femoral sheath through the fossa ovalis and extend in any direction.
- It is the most common site for Richter's hernia (*see* page 92).
- The incidence of strangulation is approximately 10 times higher than for inguinal hernias.[2]

---

2   Gallegos NC, Dawson J, Jarvis M and Hobsley M (1991) Risk of strangulation in groin hernias. *Br J Surg* **78**: 1171–3.

Risk factors

Multiparity, weight loss, previous inguinal hernia repair.

Pathogenesis

An acquired downward extension of peritoneum through the femoral canal. This process is thought to occur due to *stretching* of the femoral canal by events that raise intra-abdominal pressure, such as pregnancy and obesity. Furthermore, anatomical differences in the female pelvis may partly explain the increased incidence of femoral hernias in women.

Differential diagnosis of a 'lump in the groin'

- *Inguinal hernia*
- *Femoral hernia*
- *Hydrocele of the cord or canal of Nuck*: smooth, oval, transilluminates
- *Lipoma of the cord*: soft and lobulated with no cough impulse
- *Undescended testis*: always examine the scrotum and its contents
- *Inguinal lymphadenopathy*: often multiple and present both laterally and medially to femoral vessels
- *Saphenous varix*: easily emptied by pressure or on lying supine. There is a demonstrable 'thrill' on coughing. May be bluish in appearance
- *Ileofemoral aneurysm*: expansile mass +/– bruit
- *Psoas abscess*: usually points lateral to the femoral vessels
- *Lipoma of the fat in the femoral canal*: difficult to differentiate clinically from a femoral hernia.

Umbilical hernia

- It is common in neonates/infants but most resolve spontaneously
- Incidence in adults increases with age (uncommon before 40 years)
- There is equal incidence in males and females
- It is often irreducible.

Risk factors

Ethnicity (neonatal/infant hernia more common in black people), multiparity, obesity, intra-abdominal malignancy, ascites, and continuous ambulatory peritoneal dialysis.

Pathogenesis

Neonatal/infantile hernias are *congenital* and result from failure of closure of the umbilical cicatrix. The hernial sac protrudes through this defect into the subcutaneous tissues. *Adult* hernias are *acquired* and are a consequence of increased intra-abdominal pressure upon the umbilical cicatrix, which stretches and bulges outwards.

Incisional hernia

● Common; it may complicate up to 11% of abdominal wounds after 10 years[3]
● There is equal incidence in males and females
● It occurs most commonly in lower midline abdominal incisions but can occur at the site of any incision.

Risk factors

Poor surgical technique (incorrectly placed incision, inadequate wound closure, haematoma, necrosis, sepsis), placing drains or stomas through wounds, age, diabetes, jaundice, renal failure, obesity, malignancy, gross abdominal distension (obstruction, ascites).

Pathogenesis

Acquired weakness in the abdominal wall as a result of a surgical or accidental wound. The hernial sac protrudes through the scar. Incisional hernias represent a partial wound dehiscence where the deep layers of the abdominal wall separate, but the skin remains intact.

Complications of hernias

● *Incarceration*: contents of the hernia become stuck and cannot be reduced
● *Obstruction*
● *Strangulation*

---

3   Mudge M and Hughes LE (1985) Incisional hernia: a 10-year prospective study of incidence and attitudes. *Br J Surg* 72: 70–1.

- *Reduction en masse*: the hernial sac and its contents are reduced through the abdominal wall defect *en masse*. The contents remain compromised as they continue to be constricted by the neck of the sac
- *Spontaneous rupture* of the hernial sac (particularly incisional hernia)
- *Traumatic rupture* of the hernia following blunt trauma when the hernia is out.

Special types of hernias

Simple strangulated hernia

The blood supply to the bowel inside the hernial sac is compromised (*see* Figure 5.1).

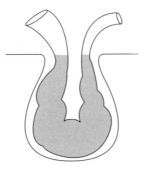

Figure 5.1   Simple strangulated hernia.

Sliding hernia

This is a type of indirect inguinal hernia in which the wall of the viscus forms part of the wall of the hernial sac. On the right side the caecum is most commonly involved, on the left the sigmoid colon (*see* Figure 5.2).

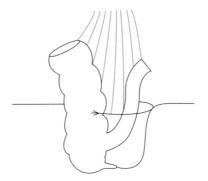

Figure 5.2   Sliding hernia.

Maydl's (W loop) hernia

There are two loops of bowel in the sac. The bowel inside the abdomen (and therefore outside the sac) is strangulated (*see* Figure 5.3).

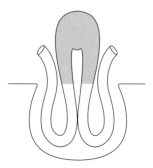

Figure 5.3 Maydl's hernia.

Richter's hernia

A knuckle of bowel is caught in the sac (and may be strangulated), but there is no obstruction (*see* Figure 5.4).

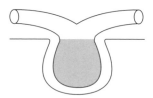

Figure 5.4 Richter's hernia.

Littre's hernia

This occurs when a Meckel's diverticulum is caught in an inguinal hernial sac.

Incarcerated/strangulated hernia

Pathogenesis

The contents of the hernia become stuck within the hernial sac. The constricting agent is usually the neck of the sac which is often fibrosed and rigid where it traverses the defect in the abdominal wall. If the hernia contains bowel, the lumen may become obstructed by the neck of the hernial sac. Strangulation occurs when the blood supply to the hernial contents is compromised causing ischaemia and necrosis.

Symptoms

- *Pain* is usually the presenting symptom; typically there is a constant ache at the site of the hernia that may be worse on movement. Severe pain occurs on initial appearance of the hernia, or if the hernia is strangulated
- A *new swelling* in the groin or elsewhere in the abdominal wall may have been noticed
- Patients with an existing hernia may complain that it is stuck
- *Abdominal distension* with *absolute constipation and/or vomiting* (suggesting obstruction).

Signs

- *Palpation* of the hernia or hernial orifice *may be painful*
- *Cough impulse may be absent*
- The hernia may be *irreducible*
- *Erythema* of the overlying skin suggests strangulation
- *Abdominal distension* and *tinkling bowel sounds* suggest *bowel obstruction.*

Investigations

- *Blood tests*: a raised WCC may suggest that the hernial contents are strangulated. CRP may also be elevated
- *AXR*: may show a knuckle of bowel at the site of the hernial orifice. Dilated loops of bowel will be evident if there is an obstruction
- *USS*: consider if there is diagnostic uncertainty.[4]

---

4   USS has a sensitivity and specificity of approximately 90% and 80% respectively for inguinal hernias. *See* Van den Berg JC, de Valois JC, Go PM and Rosenbusch G (1999) Detection of groin hernia with physical examination, ultrasound, and MRI compared with laparoscopic findings. *Invest Radiol* **34**: 739–43.

Treatment

- *Admit*
- *Nil by mouth* (NBM)
- *Analgesia*
- *Fluid resuscitation*
- If there is evidence of intestinal obstruction pass a *nasogastric tube* and *urinary catheter*
- Accurate *record of fluid balance* must be kept
- If you suspect the hernia contains compromised bowel start *empirical antibiotics* (cefuroxime and metronidazole)
- *Prepare the patient for theatre.*[5] Surgery will involve reduction of the hernial contents, resection of any strangulated bowel, and repair of the defect.[6]

---

5 If the hernia is incarcerated and there is no evidence the contents are compromised, a gentle attempt at manual reduction can be made. The patient should be observed overnight following reduction in case of complications. With groin hernias, when manual reduction is unsuccessful, lying the patient supine with the foot end of the bed elevated 30–40° may promote spontaneous reduction.

6 Mesh can be used if there is minimal contamination. *See* Wysocki A, Pozniczek M, Krzywon J and Bolt L (2001) Use of polypropylene prostheses for strangulated inguinal and incisional hernias. *Hernia* 5: 105–6.

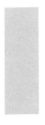

Chapter 6
Breast disorders

Breast abscess

Breast abscesses can be classified as either *lactational* or *non-lactational*.

Differential diagnosis

Inflammatory breast carcinoma (likely to be aggressive; diagnosis must not be delayed).

Lactational breast abscess

This accounts for 25% of all acute breast infections. It occurs most commonly in the first 2 months after commencing breast-feeding, but may occur on weaning.

Symptoms

Discomfort followed by a *painful swelling* of the affected breast. There is commonly a history of a *cracked nipple* or *nipple abrasion* prior to the onset of symptoms.

Signs

Tender mass in the affected segment of the breast. The overlying skin is *warm* and *erythematous*.

Causes

Organisms, usually *Staphylococcus aureus*, *Staphylococcus epidermidis*, and *Streptococci*.

Treatment

- *Aspiration*[1] ideally under *USS guidance* (send aspirate for microscopy, culture and sensitivity)
- *Antibiotics* (flucloxacillin or co-amoxiclav)
- Advise to *continue breast-feeding*/express milk in order to encourage drainage
- *Drainage through a small incision is occasionally necessary*

---

1   Thirumalakumar S and Kommu S (2004) Best evidence topic reports. Aspiration of breast abscesses. *Emerg Med J* **21**: 333–4.

- *Follow up in breast clinic* for review and possibly further aspiration
- *Perform a core biopsy if inflammation persists*, to exclude an inflammatory carcinoma.

Non-lactational breast abscess

This can occur *centrally* (most common) or *peripherally*. Central abscesses occur in younger women (mean age 32 years) and are associated with smoking in 90% of cases. Peripheral abscesses occur in older women and are associated with diabetes mellitus (DM), rheumatoid arthritis, steroids, granulomatous lobular mastitis and trauma.

Symptoms

Central abscess

- *Painful periareolar swelling*
- Associated features include *nipple discharge* and *nipple retraction* at the site of the diseased duct.

Peripheral abscess

- *Discomfort* followed by *painful swelling* in the affected part of the breast.

Signs

Central abscess

- *Periareolar inflammation +/– fluctuant mass.*

Peripheral abscess

- *Tender mass* in the affected segment of the breast. The overlying skin is *warm* and *erythematous.*

Causes

Organisms are likely to be both aerobic and anaerobic and include *Staphylococcus aureus, Enterococci*, anaerobic *Streptococci*, and *Bacteroides*.

Investigations

Investigations should be performed to exclude an inflammatory tumour and may include:

- imaging by *USS +/– mammography*
- *fine needle aspiration (FNA)/core biopsy.*

Treatment

- *Aspiration* ideally under *USS guidance* (send aspirate for microscopy, culture and sensitivity)
- *Broad-spectrum antibiotics* (e.g. co-amoxiclav or cephradine with metronidazole)
- *Drainage through a small incision is occasionally necessary*
- Patients who have a non-lactational abscess are at risk of recurrence so *definitive operative treatment* (duct excision) should be considered.

Complications

Complications include mammary duct fistula following spontaneous or surgical drainage.

Breast haematoma

This is the most common problem after breast trauma. There is ecchymosis and the presence of a mass. Most haematomas can be managed using supportive brassiere and analgesia. Iatrogenic haematomas (e.g. after a biopsy) may require surgical drainage. The decision will partly depend on how tense and painful the haematoma is and whether the biopsy was performed recently.

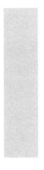

Chapter 7
Abdominal emergencies

Acute abdomen

An acute abdomen is defined as a condition associated with abdominal pain that requires surgical consultation. Remember the following points when clerking a patient with an acute abdomen:

- *ensure adequate analgesia* to relieve the patient's discomfort. This will not alter outcome or cause delay in diagnosis[1]
- *take a good history*: an accurate diagnosis can be made in the majority of cases based on history alone
- if the diagnosis is unclear and the patient is stable, a *period of observation with re-assessment* may be appropriate.

Taking an adequate history

Document the following in addition to standard history:

- *pain*:
  - location (where in the abdomen?) – *see* Figure 7.1 for common causes according to location
  - severity (out of 10)
  - time course (when did it start?)
  - nature (i.e. sharp, colicky etc)
  - radiation (which part of the body does it radiate to?)
  - exarcerbating and relieving factors
- *associated symptoms*:
  - nausea/vomiting
  - change in bowel habit
  - bleeding *per rectum*
  - loss of appetite
  - presence of a mass
  - weight loss
- in *females* enquire about *last menstrual period*
- *past medical history* including:
  - previous surgery, previous relevant outpatient examinations (e.g. barium enema, colonsocopy, oesophago-gastro-duodenoscopy (OGD), anaesthetic problems, previous admissions with the same problem
- *family history*: enquire about relevant family history (e.g. gallstones and malignancy).

Also consider medical causes of abdominal pain including pneumonia, MI, PE, and diabetes.

---

1   McHale PM and LoVecchio F (2001) Narcotic analgesia in the acute abdomen – a review of prospective trials. *Eur J Emerg Med* **8**: 131–6.

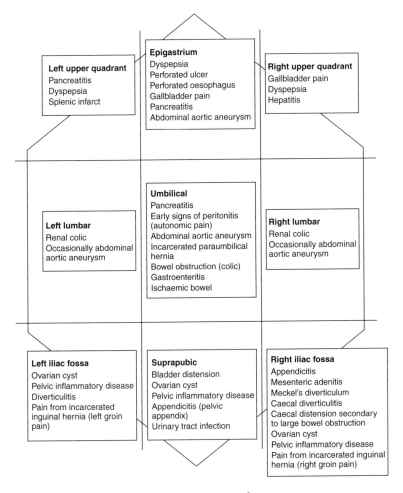

Figure 7.1 Common causes of abdominal pain.[2]

---

2   In some patients no cause can be found, but beware of making a diagnosis of 'non-specific abdominal pain' without fully investigating first.

Abdominal examination

Expose the chest and abdomen, and cover the genitalia with a towel or blanket.
Ensure that the patient is lying supine (if possible). Perform the following.

1 *General appearance*: is the patient unwell or in pain?
2 *Examine the hands*:
   - pale skin creases (anaemia)
   - peripheral cyanosis
   - koilonychia (iron-deficiency anaemia)
   - clubbing, palmar erythema, leuconychia, liver flap, Dupuytren's contracture (stigmata of liver disease)
3 *Check pulse*
4 *Examine the eyes*: look for jaundice (yellow sclerae) and anaemia
5 *Smell breath* for fetor, and examine the tongue
6 *Check jugular venous pressure (JVP)*
7 *Examine neck*[3] for lymphadenopathy
8 Then move on to the *abdomen*.

Inspection

Look for:

- *scars*
- *swellings*
- *distension*[4]
- *visible pulsations and peristalsis*
- *sinuses and fistulae*
- *distended veins.*

Palpation

Start gently and away from the site of pain whilst looking at the patient's face.
Then palpate deeper. Feel for:

- degree of *tenderness* and presence of *guarding*
- *masses*
- *splenomegaly*: begin in the right iliac fossa (RIF) and work towards the left upper quadrant (LUQ), feeling for a splenic edge as the patient breathes in

---

3 Look for Virchow's node in the left supraclavicular fossa (associated with upper GI malignancy).
4 Causes of abdominal distension are the five Fs: foetus, flatus, faeces, fat and fluid (i.e. ascites).

- *hepatomegaly*: begin in the RIF and work towards the RUQ, feeling for a hepatic edge as the patient breathes in
- *ballotable kidneys*
- *palpable bladder*
- any evidence of an *abdominal aortic aneurysm (AAA)* (expansile mass in the epigastrium, absence of femoral pulse)
- *hernial orifices*: ask the patient to cough.

Percussion

Percuss the abdomen for:

- evidence of *shifting dullness* (ascites)
- *organomegaly*
- *rebound tenderness* (suggestive of peritonism).

Auscultation

Listen for:

- *bowel sounds*
- *bruits* (femoral and splenic vessels)
- *succussion splash* (e.g. in gastric outflow obstruction).

Finally examine the external genitalia, perform a digital rectal examination, and consider a vaginal examination in females.

Abdominal masses

Remember to document the following:

- location
- shape and surface
- size
- tenderness
- consistency: cystic or solid
- pulsatile or expansile
- mobile or fixed
- can you get above or below it?
- are there any other signs associated with it?

Common abdominal masses

Epigastrium

- *Epigastric incarcerated hernia*: not reducible, tender, often containing omentum which feels firm
- *Pancreatic pseudocyst*: cystic, transmitted pulsations from aorta
- *AAA*: expansile; tender if sudden expansion or rupture
- *Carcinoma arising from stomach*
- *Left lobe of liver.*

RUQ

- *Hepatomegaly*: cannot get above it, can be smooth or craggy
- *Gallbladder*: localised mass[5]
- *Pyloric stenosis*: in children.

LUQ

- *Splenomegaly*: usually smooth, cannot get above it, classically can feel a splenic 'notch'
- *Colonic mass*: malignancy at splenic flexure.

---

5 Remember Courvoisier's law which states that if the gall bladder is palpable in the presence of jaundice the cause is unlikely to be a stone in the common bile duct (CBD). This is a useful rule but there are exceptions to it.

Right or left flank

- *Mass arising from kidney or adrenal gland.*

Central

- *Umbilical hernia*: can vary in size. May be tender and irreducible
- *Spigelian hernia*: found at the lateral border of the rectus sheath.

RIF

- *Appendix mass*: tender
- *Crohn's mass*
- *Caecal carcinoma*: may be associated with generalised distension caused by obstruction of proximal loops of small bowel
- *Psoas abscess*: may extend below the groin.

LIF

- *Diverticular mass*: usually tender
- *Colonic carcinoma*
- *Psoas abscess*: may extend below the groin
- *Faeces*: faeces are indentable.

Pelvic

- *Bladder*: dull to percussion; cannot get below it
- *Ovarian mass/cyst*
- *Fibroids*
- *Pregnancy including ectopic.*

Peritonitis

The peritoneal membrane comprises a single layer of mesothelial cells associated with supporting connective tissue. It has a visceral component that covers the intra-abdominal organs and a parietal part that faces the abdominal wall. Peritonitis is inflammation of the peritoneum. It can be *localised* or *generalised*, *primary* or *secondary*.

Localised versus generalised peritonitis

Localised peritonitis occurs when there is inflammation of a discrete area inside the abdomen. If this develops insidiously the area may become walled off from its surroundings (by omentum, adhesions and bowel loops). In generalised peritonitis there is widespread inflammation cause by a large amount of contamination. Localised peritonitis can often become generalised if the underlying pathology is left long enough.

'Peritonism'

Peritonism refers to the clinical signs of a patient with peritonitis. When any inflammation occurs inside the abdominal cavity it is initially poorly localised because the affected visceral peritoneum is innervated by the autonomic nervous system, resulting in central abdominal pain. As the inflammation progresses, the parietal peritoneum innervated by somatic nerves is affected. Pain becomes localised to the site of inflammation.

The signs of peritonitis are *guarding*, *rebound tenderness* and *board-like rigidity*. *Bowel sounds may be absent*. The patient classically has pain on movement. Rebound tenderness is best demonstrated by percussion rather than palpation (the latter technique often causes great discomfort to the patient).

Primary peritonitis

No obvious cause is found. It is usually caused by bacterial infection. Common organisms include *E. coli* and *Streptococci*. Laparotomy is often required to rule out a secondary cause. Treat primary peritonitis with broad-spectrum antibiotics.

Secondary peritonitis

There is a known cause, e.g. perforation of viscus, ischaemic or acute inflammatory processes. Treatment depends on the cause.

Gallstones

Prevalence

8% of the UK population (10% of cases are symptomatic).

Risk factors

Increasing age, female sex (female:male predominance 2:1), obesity, pregnancy, western 'meat-rich' diet, hypertriglyceridaemia, chronic liver disease, terminal ileal dysfunction (e.g. post-resection, Crohn's disease), haemolytic disease, drugs (oral contraceptive pill (OCP), clofibrate), biliary tract infection.

The old adage '*fair, fat, female, fertile, forty*' holds true in some cases.

Pathogenesis

Changes in the relative concentration of the constituents of bile (water, cholesterol, lecithin and bile salts) result in supersaturation and precipitation of cholesterol, bilirubinate, or both. Saturated bile forms microcrystals providing a nidus for subsequent stone growth. Bacteria, shed cells and foreign bodies may provide a similar nidus. In addition, *E. coli* hydrolyses conjugated bilirubin to insoluble free bilirubin that precipitates out of solution. The majority of gallstones in western countries are cholesterol based.

Biliary colic[6]

Pathogenesis

Gallstone impaction at the neck of the gallbladder obstructs the cystic duct. Sustained contraction against the blocked duct raises the pressure within the gallbladder causing pain. Pain resolves with resolution of the obstruction as a result of the stone either falling back into the gallbladder, or passing into the bile duct.

Symptoms

Gripping pain, most commonly felt in the epigastrium and RUQ (foregut pain). Typically there is a gradual increase in severity over 1–2 h but it can last longer. Pain may radiate to the right scapula and back. It is associated with *nausea* and *vomiting*. It often occurs at night, and the patient may report being woken by the pain. Attacks are often preceded by a large meal.

Signs

Uncomplicated biliary colic produces *few clinical signs*. The patient is clearly in pain and there may be an associated tachycardia. RUQ tenderness may not be a feature.

Investigations

- Approximately 10% of gallstones are visible on *AXR*
- In uncomplicated biliary colic, all other baseline investigations will usually be normal.

Differential diagnosis

- *Acute cholecystitis*: fever with localised peritonism in RUQ
- *Acute cholangitis*: fever with rigors, jaundice, RUQ pain[7]
- *Hepatitis*: liver edge may be palpable and tender
- *Primary or secondary liver tumour*

---

6 Biliary pain is not a true 'colic'. It typically lasts for several hours.
7 Known as Charcot's triad.

- *Curtis–Fitz-Hugh syndrome*[8]
- *Dyspeptic pain*: usually sharper epigastric pain
- *Pancreatitis*: tender centrally along transpyloric line
- *Right ureteric colic*: right loin pain radiating to groin +/– other urinary symptoms
- *Abdominal aortic aneurysm (AAA)*: expansile mass, pain typically radiates to the back
- *Right-sided pneumonia*
- *Ischaemic cardiac pain.*

Imaging

Ultrasound is the gold standard for detecting stones in the gallbladder with a sensitivity of >90% on first examination.

Treatment

- *Analgesia*: pethidine and diclofenac are particularly effective
- Uncomplicated attacks are usually self-limiting and do not require admission to hospital. *Admit if you are unsure of the diagnosis or if the patient is still in pain after analgesia.*

---

8 RUQ pain from ascending pelvic infection causing inflammation of the liver capsule.

Acute cholecystitis

Incidence

20% of patients admitted to hospital with biliary tract disease have acute cholecystitis.

Risk factors

95% of people with acute cholecystitis have gallstones.

Pathogenesis

Sustained high pressure in the gallbladder as a result of continued obstruction of the cystic duct, usually the result of a gallstone, reduces blood flow to the mucosa and impairs normal mucosal defences. Inflammation of the gallbladder occurs initially because of the detergent action of bile (chemical cholecystitis). Subsequent bacterial infection supervenes in 20% (enteric organisms). In severe cases, the inflammatory process causes necrosis of the gallbladder wall and perforation. Acalculous cholecystitis occurs in critically ill patients and those involved in multiple trauma. The pathogenesis remains uncertain.

Symptoms

Usually *preceded by one or more attacks of biliary colic*. Constant and severe *pain* located in the epigastrium and RUQ which is typically worse on moving. Pain may be referred to the right shoulder (if the inflammatory process involves the diaphragm). Associated symptoms include *fever*, *anorexia*, *nausea* and *vomiting*.

Signs

- *Low-grade fever*
- *Tachycardia*
- *Tenderness and guarding in RUQ* due to localised peritonism
- *Positive Murphy's sign*[9]
- Hyperaesthesia between right 9th and 11th rib posteriorly may be present (*Boas' sign*)
- There may be a *palpable mass* in the RUQ.

---

9   This is elicited by placing a hand at the costal margin in the RUQ and asking the patient to breathe in deeply. The patient experiences pain and catches their breath as the gallbladder descends and contacts the palpating hand.

Investigations

- *Elevated WCC*
- *Elevated CRP* suggesting an acute inflammatory response
- Approximately 30–40% have *deranged LFTs*. This is caused by inflammation and oedema in the biliary tract caused by a neighbouring inflamed gallbladder
- Approximately *10% of gallstones are visible on AXR*. Gas may be seen in the gallbladder wall if there is secondary infection
- *Ultrasound* is the imaging investigation of choice.

Treatment

- *Admit*
- *NBM or sips orally*
- *Analgesia*
- *Fluid resuscitation*
- *Empirical antibiotics* (ciprofloxacin/cefuroxime with metronidazole). The majority of cases respond to conservative management. Persistent pain, high-grade fever with rigors, or the presence of an ileus may indicate empyema, gangrene[10] or perforation of the gallbladder (10% of cases), and are an indication for early surgical intervention.[11]

Alternatives to surgery

Those patients who are elderly or have co-morbidity precluding a general anaesthetic may benefit from *percutaneous cholecystotomy* which can be performed under local anaesthetic.

---

10 Occurs at the fundus of the gallbladder, and is more common in those with vascular disease.

11 Historically, delayed cholecystectomy was performed unless conservative management failed. Further complications relating to gallstones occur in up to 19% of patients while waiting for cholecystectomy. To avoid additional morbidity, early laparoscopic cholecystectomy (within 72 h of onset of symptoms) is performed in many centres. There is no evidence that early laparoscopic cholecystectomy is associated with a higher conversion or complication rate than a delayed operation. *See* Lai PB, Kwong KH, Leung KL *et al.* (1998) Randomized trial of early versus delayed laparoscopic cholecystectomy for acute cholecystitis. *Br J Surg* 85: 764–7.

Mirizzi syndrome

Pathogenesis

Obstruction of the bile duct adjacent to the cystic duct caused by pressure and/or associated inflammation of a stone lodged in the cystic duct. It occurs rarely (1% of patients with cholelithiasis).

Diagnosis

Mirizzi syndrome generally has similar symptoms to other causes of obstructive jaundice including RUQ pain with recurrent bouts of cholangitis. LFTs are deranged. Investigate with USS or CT.

Treatment

This will partly depend on whether there is a cholecystocholedochal fistula (between the neck of the gallbladder and CBD), but is generally surgical with resection of the gallbladder and t-tube insertion into the CBD.

Acute cholangitis

Incidence

Approximately 10% of patients with gallstones have stones in the bile duct (choledocholithiasis) and are at risk of developing acute cholangitis.

Risk factors

Any lesion causing obstruction to the flow of bile including:

- stone in the bile duct (most common)
- tumour
- benign biliary stricture
- biliary stents and catheters
- acute pancreatitis
- endoscopic retrograde cholangiopancreatography (ERCP).

Pathogenesis

Bile stasis predisposes to bacterial infection. Bacteria, usually Gram-negative enteric aerobes, are thought to enter the biliary tree via the sphincter of Oddi. Infection can spread to involve the intrahepatic biliary tree – 'ascending cholangitis'. Septic shock may supervene as bacteria are refluxed into the circulation.

Symptoms

The classical triad of *right upper quadrant pain*, *fever with rigors*, and *jaundice* (*Charcot's triad*) is present in approximately 70%. Pain may radiate to the back and/or be referred to the right shoulder/scapula.

Signs

Presentation varies from mild symptoms to full-blown septic shock.

- Patient is *septic* and may be *shocked* – pyrexia, tachycardia, tachypnoea, warm flushed skin, hypotension
- *Jaundice*
- *Tenderness* and guarding in RUQ due to localised peritonism.

Investigations

- *Elevated WCC*
- *Elevated CRP*
- *LFTs* will usually show an *obstructive cholestatic pattern* (i.e. raised bilirubin, alkaline phosphatase (ALP) and -glutamyl transferase (-GT))
- There may be *deranged clotting* either because of DIC or biliary obstruction
- *U&Es*: renal function may be compromised if the patient is shocked
- Approximately 10% of gallstones are visible on the *AXR*. Gas may be seen within the biliary tree if the infection is caused by gas-forming organisms
- *USS* may demonstrate a stone in the bile duct with dilation of the latter.

Treatment

- *Admit*
- *NBM*
- *Analgesia*
- *Aggressive fluid resuscitation*
- *Empirical antibiotics* (ciprofloxacin and metronidazole)
- If shocked will need *central venous access* in order to monitor filling. Consult with HDU. Patients should be *catheterised* and urine output monitored closely to assess organ perfusion
- In severe cases consider urgent *ERCP* to relieve biliary obstruction.[12]

---

12 Acute suppurative cholangitis is an uncommon but serious infection of the biliary tree characterised by pain, high-grade fever with rigors, jaundice, shock, and depression of the central nervous system. It requires urgent decompression of the biliary tree usually via endoscopy. Left untreated it has a 100% mortality.

Jaundice

Yellowing of the skin, sclerae and other tissues because of excess circulating bilirubin. Clinically detectable when plasma bilirubin >30 μmol/l.

Pathogenesis

Bilirubin is produced by the breakdown of haem in the lymphoreticular system. Insoluble unconjugated bilirubin is transported to the liver bound to albumin, where it is taken up by hepatocytes and conjugated with glucuronic acid to form soluble conjugated bilirubin. It is then excreted into the gut as a constituent of bile. Bilirubin is reduced to urobilinogen in the small bowel, and 20% is reabsorbed in the terminal ileum. Urobilinogen is excreted by the liver and kidneys.

Excessive production of bilirubin, failure of uptake or conjugation by hepatocytes, or obstruction preventing excretion of bile into the gut results in jaundice.

Classification

● *Unconjugated* or *conjugated hyperbilirubinaemia* (according to type of circulating bilirubin)

or:

● *Pre-hepatic*, *hepatic*, or *post-hepatic* (according to the site of pathology, however it is often mixed).

Causes

Causes are summarised in Table 7.1.

History

Ask about the following.

● *Pain*: most commonly caused by biliary obstruction but may be liver capsular pain
● *Stool colour*: clay-coloured stools – biliary obstruction
● *Urine colour*: dark urine – biliary obstruction
● *Pruritis*: biliary obstruction
● *Weight loss*: underlying malignancy

Table 7.1   Causes of jaundice

Unconjugated hyperbilirubinaemia	Conjugated hyperbilirubinaemia
Excess production of bilirubin: Haemolytic anaemia Ineffective erythropoeisis Resorption of blood from internal haemorrhage	**Impaired hepatocyte excretion:** Membrane transport deficiency (Dubin–Johnson syndrome) Drugs, e.g. oral contraceptive pill Diffuse hepatocellular disease, e.g. hepatitis, cirrhosis
Hepatic uptake dysfunction: Gilbert's syndrome Drugs, e.g. paracetamol	**Cholestasis – intrahepatic:** Intrahepatic bile duct disease (primary biliary cirrhosis, primary sclerosing cholangitis, liver transplant)
Impaired conjugation: Physiological jaundice of newborn Genetic abnormalities of γ-GT (Crigler–Najjar syndrome) Diffuse hepatocellular disease, e.g. hepatitis, cirrhosis	**Cholestasis – extrahepatic:** Gallstones Carcinoma (ampulla, bile duct, head of pancreas) Benign biliary stricture Choledochal cyst Pancreatitis and pancreatic pseudocyst

- *Fever*: with pain and jaundice suggests cholangitis
- *Duration of symptoms*: longer duration suggests malignancy
- *Medications*: check for hepatotoxicity
- *Recreational drug use* including alcohol consumption: hepatitis
- *Sexual practice*: hepatitis
- *Recent travel*: hepatitis
- *Blood transfusion*: hepatitis
- *Recent anaesthetic*: hepatitis
- *Joint pains, malaise, anorexia*: hepatitis
- *Recent surgery*: especially biliary
- *Previous cancer*
- *Family history of jaundice*: congenital cause, e.g. Gilbert's syndrome.

Signs

- *Jaundice*
- *Stigmata of chronic liver disease*

- *Hepatomegaly*: smooth tender liver (hepatitis); irregular liver (metastases)
- *Splenomegaly* and prominent abdominal wall veins (portal hypertension)
- *Palpable gallbladder* (in the presence of jaundice suggests malignancy – Courvoisier's law)
- Rectal examination may reveal *clay-coloured stool*.

Investigations

- *Urinalysis: see* Table 7.2
- *LFTs*: these are helpful in determining the cause of jaundice. An elevated conjugated plasma bilirubin level with deranged liver enzymes may indicate a surgical cause
- *Check clotting*: prothrombin time is a good indicator of hepatic function
- *Check hepatitis serology* if it is thought that the aetiology is hepatocellular
- *AXR*: approximately 10% of gallstones are seen on plain AXR. Air may be seen in the biliary tree if a stone has recently been passed. A 'porcelain' gallbladder is associated with malignancy of the gallbladder
- *USS* will show bile duct dilatation in extrahepatic cholestasis and may reveal the cause, e.g. stone, head of pancreas lesion[13]
- *ERCP* is a useful diagnostic tool in patients with extrahepatic cholestasis. Definitive treatment may be possible at the same time
- *Liver biopsy* should be considered in the absence of duct dilatation.

Table 7.2 Changes to laboratory parameters in jaundice

	Haemolysis (pre-hepatic)	*Hepatic*	*Cholestatic (post-hepatic)*
Urine urobilinogen	↑	↑	None present
Urine bilirubin	None present	Present	Present
Serum unconjugated bilirubin	↑	↑	No change
Serum conjugated bilirubin	No change	↑	↑
Faecal urobilinogen	↑	↓	None present

---

13 Generally, extrahepatic duct dilatation alone is associated with benign disease, e.g. stones. Intrahepatic duct dilatation may suggest malignancy.

Management

- *Admit* for investigation and treatment
- *Correct clotting abnormalities* with vitamin K (10 mg i.v.)
- *Organise further imaging to confirm the cause*
- *Extrahepatic cholestasis* is a surgical problem and *requires drainage.*

Details of management for each of the specific causes of jaundice will not be discussed here.

Dyspepsia

Dyspepsia is defined as a functional disturbance of the gastrointestinal tract characterised by *abdominal discomfort, bloating and nausea.*[14]

On examination the patient has a *soft abdomen.* There may be *epigastric tenderness. Blood tests are normal* and other causes of epigastric pain have been excluded, e.g. gallbladder disease, pancreatitis or an AAA.

Dyspepsia can be divided into three categories:

- *ulcer-type dyspepsia*: primary symptom is pain
- *motility-type dyspepsia*: primary symptoms are bloating and fullness
- *reflux-type dyspepsia*: primary symptom is heartburn.

Management of dyspepsia

Patients with dyspepsia should be treated conservatively and discharged from hospital when the episode has settled. Recurring symptoms of dyspepsia in a young patient can be treated empirically with a proton-pump inhibitor such as omeprazole. This will relieve symptoms in many patients.

In most patients presenting with symptoms of dyspepsia, endoscopy will be normal.

However, older patients should have an upper GI endoscopy to exclude other pathology.

The role of *H. pylori*

H. pylori is associated with peptic ulcer disease. Eradication of *H. pylori* can also relieve symptoms of dyspepsia.[15]

---

14 Previously it was believed that all dyspeptic pain was attributable to peptic ulcer disease. Following the introduction of endoscopy it was noticed that the majority of these patients did not have ulceration.

15 Some clinicians believe that all patients with dyspepsia should be tested for *H. pylori* and treated accordingly.

Perforated peptic ulcer

There has been a decrease in the incidence of duodenal ulceration over the last few decades but the incidence of gastric ulceration remains stable. Approximately 50% of patients with perforation will have a previous history of peptic ulcer disease. Mortality following perforation is 5–10%.

Risk factors

- Family history
- Male (ratio male:female 2:1)
- Age (duodenal ulcer (DU) 35–45 years, gastric ulcer (GU) older age group)
- *H. Pylori* infection (present in 90–100% DU, and 70% GU)
- Smoking
- Alcohol
- Drugs (NSAIDS, steroids)
- Burns
- Gastrin hypersecretion (Zollinger–Ellison syndrome)
- Hyperparathyroidism.

Pathogenesis

This is not well understood. There is an imbalance between production of damaging agents (acid and pepsin), and mucosal defences of the stomach and duodenum. There is some evidence that duodenal ulceration is largely the result of overproduction of acid, whereas gastric ulceration results from failure of mucosal defences. Perforation with leakage of gastric and duodenal contents into the peritoneal cavity causes chemical peritonitis. Subsequent bacterial peritonitis supervenes.

Symptoms

Sudden onset of severe epigastric pain due to localised peritoneal irritation. Subsequently, the pain may become more generalised. The pain is made worse by moving or coughing. Pain may occasionally radiate to the shoulder tip because of irritation of the diaphragm.

Signs

- Patient is *distressed*
- Patient *may prefer to lie still* so as not to exacerbate the pain
- Initially *tender* with *guarding and rebound in the epigastrium.* Tenderness may subsequently become *generalised* (i.e. peritonitis)
- *Bowel sounds* may be *reduced or absent* as peritonitis develops
- Signs of *systemic sepsis* will develop over time.

Investigations

- *Elevated WCC*
- *Elevated CRP*
- *Amylase* may be mildly *elevated*
- *In severe sepsis* there may be *deranged LFTs/clotting*
- *Erect CXR* will demonstrate free air under the diapragm in approximately 75% of cases. Sitting the patient upright for 10 min before the X-ray or gastric insufflation via a nasogastric tube may increase the detection rate. A *lateral decubitous X-ray* will demonstrate free air in many cases if the patient is too unwell to tolerate an erect chest X-ray
- *USS* may be more sensitive than erect CXR in detecting a pneumo-peritoneum.[16] However this is not routinely performed.

Treatment

- *Admit*
- *NBM*
- *Analgesia*
- *Fluid resuscitation*
- *Correct any electrolyte imbalance*
- A *NG tube* should be inserted and aspirated regularly
- A *urinary catheter* should be inserted and urine output monitored hourly
- Empirical *antibiotics* (cefuroxime and metronidazole)
- A *central venous catheter* may be necessary

---

16 Chen SC, Yen ZS, Wang HP *et al.* (2002) Ultrasonography is superior to plain radiography in the diagnosis of pneumoperitoneum. *Br J Surg* **89**: 351–4.

- After resuscitation the patient should *proceed to theatre* without delay for surgical repair of the perforation and peritoneal lavage[17,18]
- *Post-operative H. pylori eradication*, and PPI treatment.

Occasionally peptic ulcer perforation is treated conservatively in patients with significant co-morbidity. In the event of deterioration, surgery may be unavoidable.

---

17 Risk factors for poor outcome after surgery include age, co-morbidity, resection surgery and delay in reaching theatre. *See* Kujath P, Schwandner O and Bruch HP (2002) Morbidity and mortality of perforated peptic gastroduodenal ulcer following emergency surgery. *Langenbecks Arch Surg* **387**: 298–302.
18 Perforated gastric ulcers should be biopsied at surgery to exclude malignancy.

Oesophageal perforation

This is uncommon and has a high mortality.

Causes

- Most common cause is *iatrogenic*[19] (e.g. mechanical perforation during endoscopy)
- *Post-operatively* (e.g. Nissen fundoplication)
- *Caustic injury* (sodium hydroxide or button batteries)
- *Boerhaave syndrome.*[20]

Pathogenesis

There is leakage of oesophageal contents into the mediastinum, resulting in mediastinitis and systemic toxicity.

Symptoms

- Sudden onset of *epigastric/chest pain* radiating through to the back[21]
- *Fever*
- In Boerhaave syndrome there is a history of *vomiting*.

Signs

- *Pyrexia*
- *Shock/sepsis*
- *Surgical emphysema*
- '*Hamman's' sign* (crunching on auscultation due to air in the mediastinum).

---

19 Instrumental perforation occurs most commonly at the cervical level, mid-oesophagus and just proximal to a stricture that is being dilated. Patients with achalasia who are undergoing balloon dilatation of the lower oesophageal sphincter are also at increased risk. Perforation may occur some days after the procedure.
20 Perforation in the lower oesophagus caused by vomiting against a closed cricopharyngeus.
21 Cervical perforation is associated with pain on neck movement.

Differential diagnosis

- *MI*
- *Perforated peptic ulcer*
- *Ruptured AAA*
- *Dissecting thoracic aorta*
- *Pancreatitis*
- *Gallbladder pain.*

Investigations

- *Elevated WCC*
- *Elevated CRP*
- *U&Es* may be deranged (due to vomiting)
- *In severe sepsis* there may be *deranged LFTs/clotting*
- *Arterial blood gases* may show a *metabolic acidosis*
- *CXR* (look for subcutaneous emphysema, mediastinal widening, hydropneumothorax and pleural effusions)
- *Water-soluble contrast swallow or CT scan.*

Treatment

- *Admit*
- *NBM*
- *Analgesia*
- *Fluid resuscitation*
- *Broad-spectrum antibiotics* (e.g. cefuroxime and metronidazole)
- *Urinary catheter.* Monitor urine output hourly
- Consider whether the patient should have *surgery* or *conservative management*.

Conservative management

Conservative management is appropriate for cervical perforations, in those with significant co-morbidity or for small localised perforations. Parenteral or jejunal feeding will be necessary. If the patient deteriorates, surgery may be appropriate.

In some cases, oesophageal stenting may be successful, e.g. in those with oesophageal malignancy.

Surgical management

Surgical management is almost always necessary in Boerhaave syndrome. Surgery involves repair of the perforation and insertion of drains into the mediastinum. Oesophageal resection may be necessary.

Acute pancreatitis

An acute inflammatory process of the pancreas. Mortality has remained at 10–15% over the last 20 years.

Incidence

Approximately 1 in 1000. M > F.

Aetiology

- *Gallstones*: most common (45–50%)
- *Alcohol (35%)*
- *Drugs*
- *Trauma*
- *Post-ERCP*
- *Hypercalcaemia*
- *Infection*: parasites, mumps, rubella
- *Ischaemia*
- *Hyperlipidaemia.*

Pathophysiology

Proteolytic destruction of pancreatic substance, necrosis of blood vessels with haemorrhage, and associated inflammatory reaction. Activation of trypsinogen (into trypsin) is thought to be an important triggering event in the process.

Symptoms

- *Upper abdominal pain* classically radiating through to the back (in 90% of cases)[22]
- *Nausea or vomiting* (in 70% of cases)
- *Fever* (in 70% of cases)
- *Distension*
- *Dyspnoea* (in 20% of cases).

---

22 Rarely a patient may have no pain (e.g. in pancreatitis due to ischaemia following hypothermia or cardiopulmonary bypass).

Signs

- *Pyrexia*
- *Tachycardia*
- *Shock*
- *Epigastric tenderness* +/– rebound
- *Bluish discoloration in the flank* (Grey–Turner's sign) or *periumbilical area* (Cullen's sign), due to spread of blood retroperitoneally[23]
- *Other signs depend on the cause* (e.g. jaundice with gallstone pancreatitis).

Investigations

- *Elevation of serum amylase*[24]: four times normal is generally diagnostic
- *Urinary amylase*: useful if serum amylase is equivocal
- *Serum lipase* is more sensitive and specific than amylase: useful in delayed presentation when serum amylase has returned to normal
- *Other blood tests*: FBC, U&Es, LFTs,[25] CRP, lactate dehydrogenase (LDH), glucose (*see* prognostic indicators, below)
- *Erect CXR*
- *Abdominal film* may reveal a sentinel loop of distended small bowel. The hepatic flexure of the colon may be distended (colon 'cut-off' sign). Calcification of the pancreas indicates chronic inflammation
- *Arterial blood gases* may reveal hypoxia, metabolic acidosis
- *Ultrasound scanning* is the most sensitive method of evaluating the biliary tree, and may indicate aetiology. Views of the pancreas can be limited when there is bowel gas overlying the pancreas
- *Contrast-enhanced CT scanning* allows better visualisation of retroperitoneal structures, and may have a role in predicting outcome. CT scanning is especially useful in diagnosing later complications (*see* below), such as necrosis and pseudocyst formation.[26]

---

23 Associated with severe necrotising pancreatitis.
24 The amylase levels rise within the first 12 h, and then fall to normal within 48–72 h. However the following can also cause a rise in amylase: *small bowel obstruction, gallbladder disease including cholangitis, mesenteric ischaemia, renal insufficiency,* or *macroamylasaemia*. Amylase levels do not predict the severity of pancreatitis.
25 An elevated AST and/or ALT may indicate a diagnosis of gallstone pancreatitis, even in the absence of stones on sonography. *See* Tenner S, Dubner H and Steinberg W (1994) Predicting gallstone pancreatitis with laboratory parameters: a meta-analysis. *Am J Gastroenterol* **89**: 1863–6.
26 Dynamic CT pancreatography can identify pancreatic perfusion defects suggestive of necrosis.

Differential diagnosis

- *Acute cholecystitis*
- *Perforated duodenal ulcer/lower oesophagus*
- *Ruptured AAA*
- *Any other cause of peritonism*
- *Idiopathic hyperamylasaemia.*

Prognostic indicators and risk stratification

Numerous prognostic scoring systems are used including *Ranson's* and *Glasgow* criteria, *CRP*, *APACHE II* (Acute Physiology and Chronic Health Evaluation) and contrast-enhanced *CT scoring.*[27]

Ranson's criteria[28]

The parameters in Table 7.3 are measured on presentation and at 48 h. Mortality rises with the number of positive criteria (3–4 = 20% mortality, and greater than 6 = 90% mortality).

Table 7.3 Ranson's criteria

On presentation	At 48 h
Age > 55 years	Haematocrit > 10% rise
WCC > 16000/mm³	BUN > 1.8 ml/l rise
Glucose > 11.2 mmol/l	Ca^{2+} < 2.0 mmol/l
Lactate dehydrogenase > 350 U/l	Base deficit > 4 mmol/l
Aspartate aminotransferase (AST) > 250 U/l	Fluid loss > 6 l

27 Balthazar EJ, Robinson DL, Megibow AJ and Ranson JH (1990) Acute pancreatitis: value of CT in establishing prognosis. *Radiology* 174: 331–6.

28 Ranson's criteria may have poor predictive power. *See* De Bernardinis M, Violi V, Roncoroni L *et al.* (1999) Discriminant power and information content of Ranson's prognostic signs in acute pancreatitis: a meta-analytic study. *Crit Care Med* 27: 2272–83.

Glasgow scoring system

This should be performed on admission and repeated at 48 h. Three or more positive criteria from Table 7.4 suggest severe pancreatitis.

Table 7.4   Glasgow scoring system

Parameter	Finding
Age	>55 years
White cell count	>15 × 10^9/l
Glucose	>10 mmol/l
Urea	>16 mmol/l
PaO$_2$	<60 mmHg
Calcium	<2 mmol/l
Albumin	<32 g/l
Lactate dehydrogenase	>600 U/l
AST	>100 U/l

CRP

A CRP > 150 mg/l at 48 h after onset of symptoms is an independent predictor of severity.

Treatment

Treatment is essentially supportive.

- *NBM*[29]
- *Analgesia*
- *Oxygen*
- *Fluid resuscitation*
- *NG tube* in those with ileus or vomiting
- *Urinary catheter* with hourly urine measurements
- *Stop any possible precipitating causes* such as drugs
- *Consider HDU/ITU* in severe cases
- *Consider broad-spectrum* antibiotics in severe cases[30]

---

29 Enteral nutrition (for example nasojejunal) should be considered once the patient's pain and nausea are controlled.
30 Kramer KM and Levy H (1999) Prophylactic antibiotics for severe acute pancreatitis: the beginning of an era. *Pharmacotherapy* **19**: 592–602.

- *Emergency ERCP.*[31] There is evidence that if the initial ultrasound scan shows dilatation of the common bile duct and there are deranged LFTs, then an ERCP within 72 h can reduce morbidity and mortality.

Surgery

The role of surgery is controversial. In those whose condition is deteriorating, removal of necrotic tissue coupled with drainage at laparotomy may improve prognosis. However, post-operative complications such as fistula or abscess formation can occur.

Complications of acute pancreatitis

- *Hypocalcaemia*: if tetany occurs then calcium gluconate should be given
- *Hyperglycaemia*: start an intravenous insulin infusion sliding scale
- *Necrosis*: occurs in severe pancreatitis
- *Infection*: necrotic pancreatic tissue can become secondarily infected. Mortality increases substantially if this occurs. Diagnosis of infected necrosis may be achieved by CT-guided biopsy. Percutaneous pancreatic necrosectomy may have a role. If abscess formation occurs, then treatment will involve percutaneous drainage
- *Pseudocyst formation*: this is a collection of fluid surrounded by granulation tissue (i.e. no true wall) and classically develops 4 weeks after the episode of pancreatitis. USS or CT will confirm the diagnosis. Small cysts tend to resolve. Larger cysts may require drainage either percutaneously, endoscopically or operatively
- *Small bowel obstruction*: usually resolves once the inflammation settles
- *Haemorrhage*: usually from the splenic artery which lies in close proximity. Mortality is high.

Further treatment

Ideally cholecystectomy should be performed within 2 weeks of admission if gallstones are the cause of pancreatitis.[32] Furthermore, all patients who have pancreatitis should be followed up in clinic in order to detect complications such as pancreatic pseudocysts.

---

31 ERCP should only be performed routinely if the likely aetiology is gallstones. *See* Gregor JC, Ponich TP and Detsky AS (1996) Should ERCP be routine after an episode of 'idiopathic' pancreatitis? A cost–utility analysis. *Gastrointest Endosc* **44**: 118–23.
32 Working Party of the British Society of Gastroenterology, Association of Surgeons of Great Britain and Ireland, Pancreatic Society of Great Britain and Ireland and Association of Upper GI Surgeons of Great Britain and Ireland (2005) UK guidelines for the management of acute pancreatitis. *Gut* **54** (Suppl 3): iii1–9.

Chronic pancreatitis

This is irreversible chronic inflammation of the pancreatic acini.

Causes

- *Alcohol* (70%)
- *Autoimmune disease*
- *Hypertriglyceridaemia*
- *Hyperparathyroidism*
- *Pancreas divisum*
- *Idiopathic.*

Diagnosis

Features include:

- *recurrent episodes of acute pancreatitis*
- *chronic pain*
- *steatorrhoea*
- *weight loss*
- *diabetes mellitus.*

Investigations

- As for acute pancreatitis[33]
- *AXR*: may show calcification of the pancreas and/or a 'sentinel loop' of bowel
- *CT*: has a sensitivity of 75–90%
- *ERCP*: remains the gold standard but has associated morbidity
- *MRCP* (magnetic resonance cholangiopancreatography) *and endoscopic ultrasound* are increasingly being used
- *Pancreatic function tests*: endocrine (fasting glucose, glucose tolerance test); exocrine (secretin–cholecystokinin test).

---

33 A normal serum amylase does not exclude acute pancreatitis in these patients.

Treatment

- *Analgesia*: many of these patients require opiates (e.g. regular pethidine or morphine sulphate tablets (MST)). Consider a local anaesthetic coeliac plexus block in those with refractory pain
- *Treat the cause*: e.g. advise on alcohol abstinence
- *Diet*: avoidance of dietary fat may help symptoms
- *Pancreatic enzyme supplementation*:[34] e.g. 'Creon'.

---

34 Administer with PPI.

Acute appendicitis

Incidence

80 000 patients per annum in the UK.

Aetiology

Diet (lack of fibre), genetic factors, poor hygiene. Possible infectious aetiology (viral).

Pathophysiology

Inflammation of the appendiceal wall causes venous congestion which impairs arterial inflow leading to ischaemia and gangrene. Organisms from the lumen then enter the devitalised wall. Perforation may occur.

Symptoms

- *Pain* is the most common initial symptom. It is initially central and diffuse, due to early obstruction and dilation of the appendix (visceral pain). As the serosa of the appendix becomes involved, the pain moves to the RIF and is sharper (due to peritoneal irritation). Typically the pain is worse on movement
- *Anorexia*
- *Nausea and vomiting*
- *Fever*
- Other symptoms may include *diarrhoea* (irritation of the rectum), *testicular pain* and *dysuria* (irritation of the bladder).

Signs

- *Pyrexia*
- *Flushed appearance*
- *Dry/coated tongue with foetor*
- *Tenderness and guarding in the RIF*[35]
- Palpation of the LIF may produce pain in the RIF (*Rovsing's sign*)

---

35 The position of the appendix has an influence on the signs and symptoms. If the appendix is retrocaecal signs may be lateral to *McBurney's point* (which lies one-third of the way between the anterior superior iliac spine and the umbilicus). If the appendix lies over the pelvic brim, then vomiting and diarrhoea are more common and rectal examination may reveal tenderness. If the appendix lies in front of the ileum (i.e pre-ileal), then the signs are very obvious, whereas a postileal appendix may have few signs (*see* Figure 7.2).

- Passive extension of hip increases pain (*Psoas stretch sign*)
- There may be an *appendix mass*
- *Rectal* and *vaginal examination* are usually *normal*.

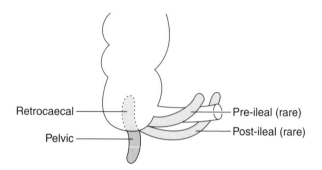

Retrocaecal ——————

Pelvic ——————

—————— Pre-ileal (rare)

—————— Post-ileal (rare)

Figure 7.2   Variable positions of the appendix.

Differential diagnosis

- *Meckel's diverticulitis*: virtually indistinguishable and must be looked for at surgery if the appendix appears normal
- *Mesenteric adenitis*[36]
- *Diverticulitis*
- *Ectopic pregnancy*
- *Crohn's disease* (diarrhoea may be a prominent feature)
- *Ovarian pathology* (torsion of cyst/ovary, mittelschmerz)
- *Pelvic inflammatory disease* (vaginal discharge)
- *Cholecystitis*
- *Constipation*
- *Non-specific abdominal pain.*

Investigations

- *FBC*: approximately 90% of patients have a raised WCC

---

36 Appendicitis is rare in preschool children and can present late. Mesenteric adenitis in contrast is common in young children and is associated with a recent viral infection (ask about upper respiratory tract infection (URTI)/recent illness). Symptoms are often more vague and vomiting is rarely a feature.

- *Elevated CRP*[37]
- *Urine dipstick and pregnancy test* on females of child-bearing age
- *AXR* is usually not helpful.

If there is diagnostic uncertainty consider:

- *'active' observation:*[38] with regular clinical review
- *USS:*[39] useful for excluding other pelvic conditions; may also demonstrate a swollen inflamed appendix or mass
- *CT:* particularly in the elderly to exclude caecal pathology[40]
- *laparoscopy.*

Treatment

- *Admit*
- *NBM*
- *Analgesia*
- *Fluid resuscitation*
- *Broad-spectrum i.v. antibiotics* reduce the incidence of post-operative wound sepsis. Use co-amoxiclav and metronidazole adjusted to weight[41]
- *Surgery.*

Surgery

Options for surgery are as follows.[42]

1 *Open appendicectomy:* through a Lanz or Grid-iron incision

---

37 CRP has medium diagnostic accuracy, and is inferior to white cell count. *See* Hallan S and Asberg A (1997) The accuracy of C-reactive protein in diagnosing acute appendicitis. *Scand J Clin Lab Invest* **57**: 373–80.

38 There is no increase in perforation rate or length of stay in hospital by pursuing a policy of 'active observation' over the first 24 h. *See* Jones PF (2001) Suspected acute appendicitis: trends in management over 30 years. *Br J Surg* **88**: 1570–7.

39 Orr RK, Porter D, Hartman D (1995) Ultrasonography to evaluate adults for appendicitis: decision making based on meta-analysis and probabilistic reasoning. *Acad Emerg Med* **2**: 644–50.

40 In older patients 'appendicitis' may be the presenting feature of a caecal carcinoma distending the appendix base.

41 Anderson BR, Kallehave FL and Anderson HK (2003) Antibiotics versus placebo for prevention of postoperative infection after appendicectomy. *Cochrane Database Syst Rev* **2**: CD001439.

42 Whether laparoscopy or open appendicectomy is 'better' is unclear at the present time, with no firm conclusions so far from the literature. The laparoscopic method appears to improve recovery time, but may take longer to perform, depending on the skill of the surgeon.

2 *Laparoscopic appendicectomy*: particularly in female patients where ovarian pathology may be a possibility.

Complications of acute appendicitis

● *Perforation with peritonitis*: those at highest risk of perforation include:
  − very young patients (less than 2 years)
  − elderly patients
  − diabetic patients (due to neuropathy)
  − patients taking steroids
● *Appendix mass/abscess*: this complicates a localised perforation when pus cannot enter the peritoneal cavity because of adherent omentum. Treatment may be conservative if systemically well (with antibiotics +/− interval appendicectomy) or immediate surgery.

Meckel's diverticulum

A diverticulum which is a congenital remnant of the vitello-intestinal duct. It may contain ectopic gastric mucosa.

It is:

- found in 2% of patients
- found 2 feet from the ileocaecal valve on the anti-mesenteric side of the ileum
- 2 inches long
- twice as frequent in males as in females.

Meckel's diverticulum is often identified incidentally. In adults an incidentally discovered, asymptomatic Meckel's should probably be left in place.[43]

A Meckel's diverticulum may present with:

- *diverticulitis*: which mimics appendicitis[44]
- *peptic ulceration*
- *haemorrhage*: the most common cause of lower GI haemorrhage in paediatric patients
- *intussusception*: acts as a leadpoint
- *obstruction*: caused by a band between the diverticulum and the umbilicus.

---

43 Leijonmarck CE, Bonman-Sandelin K, Frisell J and Raf L (1986) Meckel's diverticulum in the adult. *Br J Surg* 73: 146–9.
44 When carrying out an appendicectomy always check the ileum in a patient with a normal appendix, to exclude an inflamed Meckel's diverticulum.

Diverticular disease

Definitions

- *Diverticulum*: an outpouching in the wall of the gut
- *Diverticulae*: *plural*
- *Diverticulosis*: the presence of diverticulae
- *Diverticulitis*: inflammation within the diverticulum
- *Diverticular disease*: diverticulae causing symptoms.

Incidence

Common in the west; 50% aged over 70 years have diverticulosis.

Risk factors

Age, diet (lack of fibre), genetic factors, constipating medication, smoking.[45]

Pathophysiology

Diverticulae are thought to arise from increased pressure within the lumen of the bowel. They occur at weak areas between taeniae where vessels perforate through the submucosal layer. The sigmoid colon is most commonly affected.[46]

Complications of diverticulae

- *Inflammation (diverticulitis)*
- *Abscess formation*
- *Perforation*
- *Fistula formation*
- *Obstruction*
- *Bleeding.*

---

45 Smoking is an independent risk factor for complications of diverticular disease. *See* Papagrigoriadis S, Macey L, Bourantas N and Rennie JA (1999) Smoking may be associated with complications in diverticular disease. *Br J Surg* **86**: 923–6.

46 However, right-sided colonic diverticulae can occur. They are especially common in the young and in patients from Asian countries.

Inflammation (diverticulitis)

Inspissation of stool within the neck of a diverticulum causes inflammation and possible microscopic rupture. A commonly used classification of the severity of diverticulitis is shown in Box 7.1.

Box 7.1   Modified Hinchey classification of diverticulitis

- *Stage I*: pericolic abscess
- *Stage IIa*: distant abscess amenable to percutaneous drainage
- *Stage IIb*: complex abscess associated with/without fistula
- *Stage III*: generalised purulent peritonitis
- *Stage IV*: faecal peritonitis.

Symptoms

- *Pain*: pain is usually localised in the left iliac fossa
- *Fever*: this can be periodic (especially if there is an abscess).

Other symptoms may include:

- *nausea and vomiting*
- *diarrhoea*
- *constipation.*

Signs

- *Pyrexia* which may be swinging
- *Tenderness in the LIF. Guarding* and *rebound tenderness* suggest peritonitis
- Presence of a *mass*
- *Rectal examination* may reveal tenderness on the left side or a mass.

Investigations

- *FBC*: there may be a raised WCC
- *Elevated CRP*
- *Urinary dipstick* may be positive for leucocytes or blood
- *Erect CXR + plain AXR* are usually unhelpful but are commonly ordered to exclude complications, e.g. perforation / obstruction
- *USS* may demonstrate an abscess

- CT is the imaging modality of choice to detect diverticulitis and its complications.[47] However not all patients admitted with diverticulitis will require a CT.

Differential diagnosis

- *Colorectal cancer*
- *Appendicitis*
- *Crohn's disease*: diarrhoea is a prominent symptom
- *Pelvic inflammatory disease*
- *Colitis*: ulcerative colitis (UC)/ischaemic/infective
- *Diverticular pain* (i.e. symptoms from existing diverticulae but with no inflammation)
- *AAA*
- *Acute epiploic appendagitis.*[48]

Treatment

- *Admit*
- *NBM* but allow fluids when clinically better
- *Analgesia*
- *Fluid resuscitation*
- *Broad-spectrum i.v. antibiotics* (cefuroxime 750 mg i.v. tds and metronidazole 500 mg tds)
- *Review regularly* and *check bloods daily.*

More than half of all patients treated for a first episode of diverticulitis will recover and have no further problems in the future.[49]

---

47 Eggesbo HB, Jacobsen T, Kolmannskog F, Bay D and Nygaard K (1998) Diagnosis of acute left-sided colonic diverticulitis by three radiological modalities. *Acta Radiol* **39**: 315–21.

48 This is an uncommon cause of abdominal pain. It occurs from inflammation of an appendix epiploica.

49 Many surgeons advocate definitive elective surgery in young patients who have had two episodes of diverticulitis. However, this belief is now being challenged. A recent study has shown that after an episode of diverticulitis, the risk of an individual requiring an urgent Hartmann's procedure is one in 2000 patient-years of follow-up. *See* Janes S, Meagher A and Frizelle FA (2005) Elective surgery after acute diverticulitis. *Br J Surg* **92**: 133–42. Patients with significant co-morbidity may be successfully managed with long-term antibiotic prophylaxis and cessation of NSAIDs.

Abdominal abscess

This can develop from diverticulitis. If suspected, CT is the imaging modality of choice. It may be amenable to percutaneous drainage under antibiotic cover. Surgical drainage may be necessary.

Perforation

Peritonitis occurs following rupture of an inflamed diverticulum or of a previously contained abscess. Faecal peritonitis may result.

Fistula formation

Colovesical fistula is the most common type of fistula associated with diverticulitis. It is more common in males. Patients present with pneumaturia, faecaluria, and recurrent UTIs. Colorectal carcinoma can also cause this type of fistula. Further investigations should be organised including a CT with rectal contrast. Surgery may be required.

Colovaginal fistula formation occurs more commonly in those who have previously had a hysterectomy. Patients present with purulent or faeculent vaginal discharge.

Symptoms and signs

Sudden increase in pain associated with *systemic toxicity* and signs of *localised or generalised peritonitis.*

Investigations

- *As for diverticulitis*
- *LFTs* and *clotting* may be deranged (because of portal pyaemia)
- *Arterial blood gases* may reveal a metabolic acidosis
- *Erect CXR* may reveal free air under the diaphragm.

Treatment

- *As for diverticulitis*
- *Prepare the patient urgently for theatre.*[50]

Obstruction

This is frequently difficult to differentiate from malignant obstruction (*see* 'Large bowel obstruction', page 155).

Diverticular bleeding

See 'Lower gastrointestinal haemorrhage', page 172.

---

50 Surgery involves laparotomy, washout and resection of the affected section of colon (usually the sigmoid colon). This will usually necessitate a Hartmann's procedure. However, a recent systematic review has reported that mortality and morbidity in patients with diverticular peritonitis who underwent primary anastomosis were not higher than for those who underwent a Hartmann's procedure. Primary anastomosis in the emergency setting should only be performed by an experienced colorectal surgeon in selective patients. *See* Salem L and Flum DR (2004) Primary anastomosis or Hartmann's procedure for patients with diverticular peritonitis? A systematic review. *Dis Colon Rectum* 47: 1953–64.

Emergencies in inflammatory bowel disease (IBD)

Crohn's disease

This can affect any part of the alimentary tract. There is chronic transmural granulomatous inflammation with skip lesions.

Ulcerative colitis

UC affects only the colon and 'spreads' proximally from the rectum. Inflammation affects only the mucosa and submucosa and is confluent.

Surgical intervention may be necessary for any of the following:

- *acute colitis*
- *toxic megacolon*
- *abscess formation*
- *fistula formation*
- *perforation*
- *obstruction*
- *haemorrhage.*

Acute colitis

Symptoms

- *Fever*
- *Frequent bloody diarrhoea*
- *Abdominal pain.*

Signs

- *Pyrexia*
- *Tachycardia*
- *Abdominal distension/tenderness.*

Acute colitis is usually managed by the gastroenterologists.

Treatment

- *Analgesia*
- *Fluid resuscitation*
- *High-dose i.v. steroids* (hydrocortisone 100 mg 6-hourly) and *immunosuppressant treatment* (e.g. cyclosporine).

Indications for surgery

- *Failure to improve clinically*[51]
- *Toxic megacolon.*[52]

Abscess formation

This usually occurs in Crohn's disease. Abscesses should be imaged using CT or USS and then drained percutaneously where possible.

Perianal abscesses in Crohn's are often complex and intimately associated with the sphincter mechanism. The patient should have an examination under anaesthesia (EUA) and drainage by an experienced colorectal surgeon. An MRI prior to surgery may provide useful information.

Fistula formation

These occur in Crohn's disease. The most common are peri-anal (60%) but entero-enteral fistulae also occur and usually involve the ileum. Surgery is usually necessary, but newer treatments may have a role (e.g. Infliximab).

Perforation

- Perforation usually occurs in the colon as a result of toxic megacolon
- Treatment involves resuscitation followed by colectomy
- Small bowel perforations in Crohn's disease are often sealed off, leading to abscess formation.

---

51 A joint decision between the surgeons and gastroenterologists is made based on clinical progress, regular FBC, CRP and the stool chart. Surgery should be considered after failure to improve after 48 h of treatment.
52 AXR should be performed daily. Dilated colon greater than 6 cm indicates megacolon.

Obstruction

This is either due to stricture formation (Crohn's disease), or malignancy (in long-standing UC).

Crohn's obstruction may be treated medically in the first instance with high-dose steroids and mesalazine. The majority will respond to medical management. However, the patient should be observed closely, and if there is any evidence of clinical deterioration, surgery should be considered.

Haemorrhage

This occurs more commonly in young patients, but severe bleeding is generally rare.

In UC, bleeding is more likely in severe disease and commonly arises from the rectum.

In Crohn's disease, bleeding occurs as a result of full-thickness ulceration eroding a blood vessel.

Abscesses

An abscess is a localised collection of pus.

Skin abscesses

Risk factors

Smoking, obesity, poor hygiene, diabetes mellitus and i.v. drug abuse.

Causative organisms

Often polymicrobial. *S. pyogenes* and *S. aureus* are the most common organisms.

Management

Incision and drainage. If sizeable, curette, irrigate and pack, allowing healing by secondary intention.[53] Beware of abscesses that might communicate with important structures (e.g. deep groin abscess near the femoral vessels). If in doubt organise an USS/CT/MRI scan to examine the configuration in greater detail.

Breast/perianal and pilonidal abscesses

See relevant sections of this book.

Intra-abdominal abscesses

Most intra-abdominal abscesses form *following perforation of a viscus.*[54] Features include *swinging pyrexia, ileus* and *leucocytosis.* If the abscess is *intraperitoneal* there may be *tenderness* over the area and a *palpable mass.*

Pelvic abscesses are best felt rectally. Retroperitoneal abscesses may not have any abdominal signs.

Management

- Diagnosis by *CT* or *USS*

---

53 Some studies have suggested that primary closure for superficial abscesses can improve the quality of healing and pain post-operatively. *See* Abraham N, Doudle M and Carson P (1997) Open versus closed surgical treatment of abscesses: a controlled clinical trial. *Aust NZ J Surg* **67**: 173–6.
54 There are more luminal organisms in the distal parts of the gut. Consequently abscesses tend to occur more commonly after colonic perforations.

- *Percutaneous drainage* by CT/USS guidance if possible
- *Send pus for microscopy culture and sensitivity* (MC&S)
- *Surgery* if percutaneous drainage is unsuccessful or not possible.

Antibiotics will not cure an abscess without drainage.

Gastrointestinal fistulae

A fistula[55] is an abnormal communication between two epithelial surfaces.

Symptoms

Symptoms depend on the site, e.g. a colovesical fistula may present with pneumaturia and recurrent urinary tract infections. However there may be no symptoms at all.

Causes

- *Bowel injury during surgery* (usually enterocutaneous)
- *Bowel inflammation*, e.g. diverticulitis, Crohn's disease,[56] and radiation enteritis
- *Malignancy*
- *Abdominal trauma.*

Fistulae may close spontaneously, but this is less likely in the following circumstances:

- high output
- distal intestinal obstruction
- poor nutritional state
- steroid treatment
- ongoing sepsis
- malignancy
- co-morbidity.

Management

- *Fluid resuscitation*
- *Correct electrolyte imbalance*
- *Treat sepsis*
- *Assess nutritional status* and consider parenteral nutrition or feeding jejunostomy below the site of the fistula
- Measures to *decrease fistula output* including reduction of oral intake and GI secretions (e.g. octreotide, PPI)

---

55 As compared to a *sinus*, which is a blind-ending tract opening onto an epithelial surface.
56 Almost half will develop a fistula during their lifetime.

- *Radiological investigations* to delineate the anatomy of the fistula, and any associated pathology, e.g. abscess, tumour. These may include a contrast enema (in the case of a colonic fistula), fistulogram or CT. Discuss with the radiologists
- *Consider specific treatment[57] for underlying disease*: e.g. surgery for malignancy/diverticular disease.

---

57 Infliximab, a monoclonal antibody against tumour necrosis factor (TNF), may be effective treatment for fistulising Crohn's disease. *See* Sands BE, Anderson FH, Bernstein CN *et al.* (2004) Infliximab maintenance therapy for fistulizing Crohn's disease. *N Engl J Med* **350**: 876–85.

Small bowel obstruction

The causes of any bowel obstruction can be classified as shown in Table 7.5.

Table 7.5   Causes of small bowel obstruction

Within the lumen	From the bowel wall	Extrinsic to the bowel
Gallstone ('gallstone ileus')[58]	Carcinoma (second commonest cause)[59]	Adhesions (most common cause)
Food	Crohn's disease	Hernia[60]
Worms (e.g. *Ascaris*)	Stricture after surgery	Volvulus
Foreign body	Ischaemic stricture	Intussusception[61]
	Radiation therapy[62]	

Symptoms

- *Central colicky abdominal pain*
- *Nausea and vomiting* (bilious or faeculent). If the obstruction is proximal vomiting is a more common feature
- *Distension*
- *Absolute constipation is often a late or absent feature.*

Signs

- *Distension*
- *Visible peristalsis*
- *Tenderness.* Signs of peritonism suggest strangulation

---

58 Results from a cholecystoduodenal fistula. Radiographically there may be evidence of air in the biliary tree. The stone impacts at the ileocaecal valve.
59 Primary malignancy of the small bowel is rare. Malignant small bowel obstruction is usually due to metastases. Treat conservatively if possible; steroids and octreotide may help.
60 The presence of a hernia may be a red herring. Raised intra-abdominal pressure due to obstruction from another pathology can cause the appearance of a hernia.
61 More common in children. Occurs in adults in association with polyps or cancers.
62 Radiotherapy can cause adhesions. Therefore treat conservatively if possible. A laparotomy for this condition may be extremely difficult with likely bowel injury during the procedure.

- *Bowel sounds may be high-pitched and tinkling or absent* (this may indicate strangulation)
- *Signs associated with the cause* (incarcerated hernia, scars from previous abdominal surgery).

Investigations

- *FBC*: raised WCC may suggest strangulation
- *U&Es*: electrolyte disturbance/renal failure due to vomiting/third-space losses
- *Consider ABGs* if the patient is unwell (metabolic acidosis may indicate strangulated bowel)
- *AXR* may show dilated small bowel loops centrally
- *CXR* to exclude the presence of free air under the diaphragm (perforation)
- *Gastrograffin follow-through*[63] or CT may be useful.

Treatment

- *Admit*
- *NBM*
- *Analgesia*
- *Fluid resuscitation*
- *Correct electrolyte disturbance*
- *Insert an NG tube. Aspirate 2-hourly*
- *Urinary catheterisation*
- *Accurate fluid balance chart*
- *Treatment of cause.*

If adhesions are the likely cause, a trial of conservative management[64] is appropriate.

---

63 Gastrograffin administration may have a therapeutic effect. Biondo S, Pares D, Mora L *et al.* (2003) Randomized clinical study of gastrograffin administration in patients with adhesive small bowel obstruction. *Br J Surg* **90**: 542–6.
64 Patients with adhesions who are treated conservatively have a shorter hospital stay but appear to have a shortened interval before re-obstruction compared to those managed operatively. *See* Miller G, Boman J, Shrier I and Gordon PH (2000) Natural history of patients with adhesive small bowel obstruction. *Br J Surg* **87**: 1240–7.

Indications for surgery

- *Evidence of strangulation or perforation*
- *Failure to improve with conservative management within 48 h*[65]
- *Obstruction due to hernia*
- *Consider early surgery in patients with an unknown cause who have no abdominal scars.*

---

65 The duration of conservative management will depend on the clinical scenario (e.g. consider longer duration in a patient who has had multiple previous laparotomies).

Large bowel obstruction

The causes of large bowel obstruction include:

- *colorectal carcinoma*[66] (most common cause accounting for ~ 65% cases)
- *diverticular disease* (10%)
- *volvulus* (5%)
- *hernia*
- *colonic intussusception*
- *strictures caused by radiation, ischaemia or old anastomosis.*

Differential diagnosis

- *Small bowel obstruction:*[67] right colonic lesions may mimic small bowel obstruction
- *Pseudo-obstruction.*

Pathophysiology

This is determined by the competency of the ileocaecal valve. If the ileocaecal valve remains competent, a closed loop of bowel is formed between the valve and the point of obstruction. Progressive colonic dilation occurs as ileal contents continue to be emptied into this 'closed loop' of obstructed colon. This results in very high intraluminal pressures. If the colon is not decompressed, the blood supply to the bowel wall becomes impaired, resulting in gangrene and perforation (commonly occurring at the caecum). In a proportion of patients the ileocaecal valve is incompetent. Consequently, reflux of colonic contents into the ileum relieves pressure within the colon, and perforation is less likely.

Symptoms

Patients usually complain of <u>colicky lower abdominal pain</u> with <u>abdominal distension</u> and <u>absolute constipation</u> (inability to pass stool or flatus *per rectum*). <u>Faeculent vomiting</u> is a late symptom and only occurs if the ileocaecal valve is incompetent. A *sharp, continuous severe pain* is indicative of *actual or*

---

66 Carcinomas of the splenic flexure are most likely to obstruct. However, a patient with obstruction is *more likely* to have a rectosigmoid tumour (since this is the most common site of colorectal malignancy).
67 A right-sided colonic malignancy should always be suspected in the elderly patient with small bowel obstruction who has not had previous abdominal surgery.

imminent perforation. There may be a background of a change in bowel habit preceding the acute event, with associated *weight loss.*

Signs

Signs may include:

- *dehydration*
- *shock*: due to sepsis following perforation
- *abdominal distension*: maximal in the flanks
- *tympanic abdomen*
- *tenderness*: particularly in the RIF – the caecum is the most common part of the colon to perforate in obstruction. Evidence of localised or generalised peritonitis suggests imminent or actual perforation
- *tinkling bowel sounds*
- *hepatomegaly*: due to metastases
- *rectal mass on DRE*: tumour or inflammatory mass.

Investigations

- *FBC*: anaemia suggests a malignant cause. *Elevated WCC* suggests an inflammatory cause *or* compromise to the bowel wall
- *U&Es*: electrolyte disturbance/renal failure due to vomiting/third-space losses
- *LFTs*: deranged LFTs raise the possibility of malignancy with liver metastases
- *ABGs*: metabolic acidosis may indicate compromise to the bowel wall
- *AXR*:[68] the colon is distended proximal to the obstruction, and collapsed distally with no gas in the rectum. If the ileocaecal valve is incompetent, dilated loops of small bowel may also be visible
- *CXR*: free air suggests perforation
- *Rigid sigmoidoscopy*: may demonstrate the obstructing lesion
- *Gastrograffin contrast enema*: can distinguish between a mechanical obstruction and pseudo-obstruction. It may also help identify the site and nature of the obstructing lesion.

---

68 Distended colon 'frames' the abdominal cavity and can be distinguished from small bowel by the haustral markings which do not traverse the entire diameter of the bowel wall.

Treatment

- *Admit*
- *NBM*
- *Analgesia*
- *Fluid resuscitation*
- *NG tube* with 2 h aspiration (if the patient is vomiting)
- *Urinary catheter* with accurate fluid balance
- If *clinically stable* and there is *no abdominal tenderness* the patient should have a *contrast enema* to determine the site of obstruction so that surgery can be planned
- If there are signs suggesting *bowel compromise* (gross colonic distension on AXR[69] and/or localised or generalised peritonitis) the patient should be given *antibiotics* (cefuroxime 1.5 g, metronidazole 500 mg i.v.), and proceed directly to *surgery after resuscitation*.

Surgical strategies for dealing with colonic obstruction

- *Right-sided lesion*: right hemicolectomy with a primary anastamosis
- *Transverse colon lesion*: extended right hemicolectomy with primary anastamosis
- *Left-sided lesion*: either a subtotal colectomy/left hemicolectomy/sigmoid colectomy with primary anastamosis or a Hartmann's procedure.[70]

Outcome of surgery

Patients presenting with large bowel obstruction due to colorectal cancer have a 15% mortality. Mortality increases with age, Dukes' staging, American Society of Anesthesiologists (ASA) grade and mode of surgery (i.e. emergency versus scheduled).[71]

---

69 A caecal diameter of >12 cm is associated with a high risk of perforation; surgery should not be delayed.

70 Resection of the lesion with formation of an end colostomy. The distal end is left as a stump. A primary anastamosis should probably only be performed by a surgeon specialising in colorectal surgery.

71 Tekkis PP, Kinsman R, Thompson MR and Stamatakis JD (2004) The Association of Coloproctology of Great Britain and Ireland study of large bowel obstruction caused by colorectal cancer. *Ann Surg* 240: 76–81.

Role of enteral stents

Stents are increasingly being used to decompress large bowel obstruction in the acute setting. The patient may then have curative surgery after appropriate preparation.[72]

---

72 There are no long-term studies as yet. In addition, there are concerns about tumour fracture and dissemination of cancer cells associated with stent insertion.

Pseudo-obstruction[73]

Pseudo-obstruction presents as large bowel obstruction (although tenderness may be less of a feature). The aetiology is functional rather than mechanical.[74]

Causes

A number of conditions can predispose the development of pseudo-obstruction:

- *electrolyte abnormalities*
- *hypothyroidism*
- *trauma*
- *cerebrovascular accident* (CVA)
- *MI*
- *sepsis* (particularly pneumonia)
- *retroperitoneal malignancy*
- *multiple sclerosis*
- *drugs*: narcotics, anti-Parkinsonian medication.

Key points in management

- *Exclude a mechanical obstruction with a contrast enema*: AXR is not diagnostic but may be helpful. Gas in the rectum if seen is a clue to the diagnosis
- *Treat the underlying cause* if possible. Supportive management (as for large bowel obstruction) is usually successful
- If there is significant dilatation consider *colonoscopic decompression* (also allows assessment of mucosal integrity) or surgical intervention (e.g. caecostomy)
- *Neostigmine infusion* may be useful in certain patients.[75]

---

73 Another name for this is Ogilvie's syndrome.
74 There is a failure of intestinal motility thought to be caused by excessive sympathetic autonomic activity and reduced parasympathetic prokinetic activity.
75 Ponec RJ, Saunders MD and Kimmey MB (1999) Neostigmine for the treatment of acute colonic pseudo-obstruction. *N Engl J Med* **341**: 137–41.

Volvulus

This is rotation of the bowel on its mesentery in an axial manner, leading to obstruction and/or necrosis.

Sigmoid volvulus

This is the most common type of volvulus (75%). The sigmoid colon rotates up to 720° either clockwise or anticlockwise. It is more common in developing countries. There is an increased incidence in patients with mental illness or dementia.

The patient presents with *abdominal distension, absolute constipation* and *pain. Vomiting* is more of a feature than in other causes of large bowel obstruction. On examination the *abdomen* is *distended* and *tympanic*. There may be an *emptiness in the left iliac fossa*.

AXR

The sigmoid colon is grossly dilated, with loss of haustrations. There is a narrowing of the rectosigmoid at the neck. Identification of the apex of the sigmoid loop under the left hemi-diaphragm is a very specific sign.[76]

Treatment

- Initial management *as for large bowel obstruction*
- Perform a *rigid sigmoidoscopy* to decompress the bowel and insert a flatus tube for at least 24 h. Flexible sigmoidoscopy if available is superior[77]
- *Surgery* is required for perforation, imminent bowel compromise or failure of endoscopic decompression. This usually involves a Hartmann's procedure or sigmoid colectomy with primary anastomosis.

In patients who have had more than one episode of volvulus, elective surgery should be considered.

---

76 Burrell HC, Baker DM, Wardrop P and Evans AJ (1994) Significant plain film findings in sigmoid volvulus. *Clin Radiol* **49**: 317–19.
77 Flexible sigmoidoscopy also allows assessment of colonic mucosa to detect infarction. *See* Brothers TE, Strodel WE and Eckhauser FE (1987) Endoscopy in colonic volvulus. *Ann Surg* **206**: 1–4.

Caecal volvulus

This is *less common than sigmoid volvulus* and occurs when a highly mobile caecum twists, because of inadequate fixation of the ascending colon during embryological development. It is more common in females and during pregnancy. The ascending colon and ileum are also involved. The diagnosis is often made late with resulting high morbidity and mortality.

Signs and symptoms are those of a distal small bowel obstruction. There may be an *emptiness in the right iliac fossa* because the caecum has moved centrally.

AXR

Classically, a comma-shaped loop of bowel is seen in the central abdomen, facing inferiorly and to the right.

Treatment

- Initial management *as for large bowel obstruction*
- *Colonoscopic decompression* is often unsuccessful
- Most patients will require *surgery*. This usually involves a right hemicolectomy or a caecopexy (+/– caecostomy).

Gastric volvulus

This is rare but potentially life-threatening. The stomach twists by more than 180° resulting in a closed loop obstruction. In most cases the stomach will twist along its long axis (organo-axial rotation). However, in one-third of cases, the stomach twists along the short axis (mesenteroaxial volvulus).

Symptoms

- *Sudden severe epigastric or chest pain*[78]
- *Upper abdominal distension*
- *Vomiting*
- *Occasionally dyspnoea.*

Investigations

- *CXR*: gas-filled viscus in the lower chest or epigastrium
- *Blood tests*: elevated WCC, amylase; occasionally raised ALP.

---

78 Chest pain is more common in those with a supradiaphragmatic volvulus.

Treatment

- *NBM*
- *Analgesia*
- *Fluid resuscitation*
- *NG tube insertion* to decompress the stomach: this may be difficult to perform
- *Prompt surgery*: involves reducing the volvulus and performing a gastropexy.

Small bowel volvulus

This is a cause of small bowel obstruction and usually results in strangulation.

Transverse colon volvulus

This is rare and the diagnosis is often made at surgery.

Ileosigmoid knotting

The ileum is knotted around a redundant twisted sigmoid.

Gynaecological causes of the acute abdomen

Ectopic pregnancy

Always remember this as a possible diagnosis in women of child-bearing age who present with an acute abdomen.

Incidence

Between 10 and 20 per 1000 pregancies.

Risk factors

Previous ectopic pregnancy, intra-uterine device (IUD), previous pelvic inflammatory disease (PID) – especially *Chlamydia* (and this probably accounts for the increasing prevalence), fertility difficulties, age, smoking.

Symptoms and signs

Lower abdominal pain +/– vaginal bleeding +/– shock.

Management

If there is a high index of suspicion or β-human chorionic gonadotrophin (β-HCG) is positive (serum β-HCG is more sensitive than urinary β-HCG), ask for an *urgent gynaecological opinion.*

Salpingitis/pelvic inflammatory disease (PID)

Caused by anaerobes, *Neisseria* and *Chlamydia.* Prevalence is increasing.

Symptoms and signs

Fever, pelvic pain, vaginal discharge. Ask about the presence of an intra-uterine contraceptive device (IUCD) and sexual history. There may be *lower abdominal tenderness*, and *tenderness* or *discharge on vaginal examination.* The diagnosis is often made at laparoscopy.

Management

Ask for a gynaecological opinion. The condition is usually treated with a 2-week course of antibiotics, e.g. doxycycline. PID can lead to formation of a tubo-ovarian abscess which will need drainage.

Ovarian pathology

Ovarian cysts can twist, rupture or bleed leading to *constant lower abdominal pain.* They may be *palpable. Diagnose by USS. Seek gynaecological assistance.*

Rupture of an ovarian follicle (Mittelschmerz) occurs in the middle of the menstrual cycle. *Pain* is the primary symptom and is caused by blood irritating the peritoneum. *Diagnosis is by USS* (shows fluid in the pouch of Douglas). The condition is self-limiting.

Endometriosis

This commonly presents in the third and fourth decades with *dysmenorrhoea, lower abdominal pain* and *other features depending on the position of the deposits* (e.g. diarrhoea associated with bowel involvement).

Upper gastrointestinal haemorrhage

Although traditionally managed by physicians, optimal management should involve a multidisciplinary team approach, especially with patients who have bleeds refractory to medical treatment.

Incidence

50 to 150 per 100 000 population in the UK. Mortality is approximately 10%.

Risk factors

Age (increased incidence with age), NSAIDs, anticoagulants, steroids, alcohol, smoking, *H. pylori* infection.

Cause

A cause of bleeding can be found in approximately 80% of patients. These include:

- *peptic ulcer* (most common cause, 35–50%)
- *gastroduodenal erosions* (8–15%)
- *oesophagitis or gastritis* (5–15%)
- *varices*[79] (5–10%)
- *Mallory–Weiss tear* (15%)
- *upper gastrointestinal malignancy* (1%)
- *Vascular malformations*[80] (5%).

Symptoms

Patients may present with *haematemesis* (vomiting fresh red blood), *coffee ground vomit* (altered black blood), or *malaena* (black tarry stools).[81] Passage of red blood *per rectum* is usually due to bleeding from the lower GI tract but can occur following upper GI bleeding. Other symptoms depend on the cause, e.g. epigastric pain with peptic ulcer disease, preceding weight loss and/or dysphagia

---

79 About half of those with known varices present with bleeding from a different GI pathology (e.g. peptic ulcer).
80 Such as Dieulafoy's lesion which is a gastric vascular malformation.
81 It may be difficult to distinguish between malaena and discoloration of the stool by iron. Malaena is black tarry stool with a characteristic offensive smell.

with upper GI malignancy. A history of recent vomiting/retching suggests a Mallory–Weiss tear.

Signs

These depend on the cause and size of bleed. They may include:

- *anaemia*
- *stigmata of chronic liver disease*
- *shock*: due to hypovolaemia
- *epigastric tenderness* (peptic ulcer disease)
- *malaena* on DRE.

Investigations

- *FBC*: low Hb + haematocrit (Hct). Platelets may be low
- *U&Es*; increased urea:creatinine ratio[82] in patients with normal renal function suggests an upper GI bleed
- *LFTs*: deranged LFTs may reflect a variceal bleed
- *Clotting*: deranged clotting may be a cause or consequence of bleeding
- *Group and save (G&S)*: cross-match 6 units blood in severe bleeding.

Non-variceal upper GI haemorrhage[83]

Acute management

The protocol for managing upper gastrointestinal bleeding is summarised in Figure 7.3.

- *Admit*
- *NBM*
- *Insert two large-bore cannulas*
- *Fluid resuscitation*. If the patient has a severe bleed (active haematemesis and/or haematemesis with shock), or a Hb < 10 g/dl give O –ve blood but preferably cross-matched blood if available
- *Urinary catheter* with accurate fluid balance
- *Correct clotting* if deranged

---

82 Due to the 'protein meal' effect of blood digestion.
83 British Society of Gastroenterology Endoscopy Committee (2002) Non-variceal upper gastrointestinal haemorrhage: guidelines. *Gut* **51** (Suppl 4): iv1–6.

- *Commence PPI*[84] *empirically* (80 mg omeprazole i.v. stat, followed by 8 mg/h infusion for 72 h in severe bleeds)
- *Consider central venous access*
- *Urgent OGD* if the patient has a severe bleed, otherwise it may be performed within 24 h of admission.

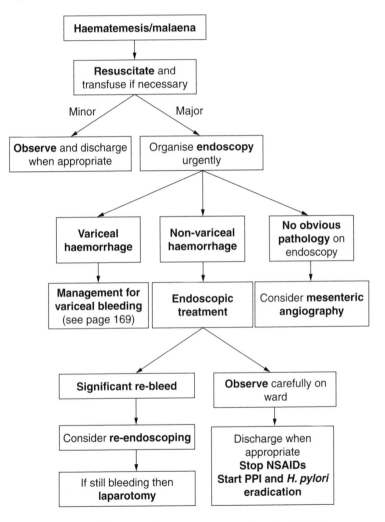

Figure 7.3 Protocol for managing an upper gastrointestinal bleed.

---

84 Treatment is intended to maintain gastric pH at >6 (the stability of a blood clot is reduced in an acidic environment).

Endoscopy

Endoscopy is useful in the acute setting to:

- define the cause of haemorrhage (and direct management)
- treat the cause (shown to improve prognosis in severe bleeds)
- determine prognosis.

The stigmata of recent haemorrhage and associated re-bleed rates are shown in Table 7.6.

Table 7.6   Modified Forrest classification for upper GI haemorrhage

Class	Endoscopic findings	Re-bleed rate (%)
Ia	Spurting artery	80–90
Ib	Oozing haemorrhage	10–30
IIa	Non-bleeding visible vessel	50–60
IIb	Adherent clot	25–35
IIc	Ulcer base with black spot sign	0–8
III	Clean base	0–12

Risk stratification

Independent factors which accurately predict a patient's risk of re-bleeding and death following an upper GI haemorrhage comprise increasing age, co-morbidity, shock, and endoscopic findings. These factors can be scored as shown in Table 7.7.

A score of 3 or less = low risk; a score of >8 = high risk. Maximum score = 11.

Indications for surgery

Urgent surgery is indicated if there is:

- *persistent hypotension despite adequate resuscitation* (6 unit transfusion in patients >60 years, 8 unit transfusion in patients <60 years)
- *bleeding during endoscopy that prevents adequate visualisation or control.*

Patients who re-bleed following a period of clinical stability should undergo repeat endoscopy to allow one further attempt at endoscopic treatment.[85] Surgery is indicated for most patients if re-bleeding occurs for a second time.

---

85 Lau JYW, Sung JJL, Lam T *et al.* (1999) Endoscopic retreatment compared with surgery in patients with recurrent bleeding after initial endoscopic control of bleeding ulcers. *N Engl J Med* **76**: 751–6.

Table 7.7   Rockall scoring system for upper GI haemorrhage

	Score			
	0	*1*	*2*	*3*
Age (years)	<60	60–79	>79	
Shock	No shock	Tachycardia (pulse >100/min)	Tachycardia (pulse >100/min); hypotension (systolic pressure <100 mmHg)	
Co-morbidity	None		Ischaemic heart disease; cardiac failure	Renal failure; liver failure; disseminated malignancy
Endoscopic diagnosis	Mallory–Weiss tear or no lesion *and* no stigmata of recent haemorrhage	All other diagnoses except malignancy	Upper GI malignancy	
Stigmata of recent haemorrhage	None or dark spot only		Blood in upper GI tract; adherent clot; visible/spurting vessel	

Variceal bleeding[86]

This is defined as bleeding from an oesophageal or gastric varix at the time of endoscopy *or* the presence of large oesophageal varices with blood in the stomach and no other recognisable cause of bleeding.

86 R Jalan and PC Hayes (2000) UK guidelines on the management of variceal haemorrhage in cirrhotic patients. British Society of Gastroenterology. *Gut* **46** (Suppl 3–4): III1–III15.

Risk factors

All causes of portal hypertension.[87]

Acute management of bleeding oesophageal varices

- *Initial management as for non-variceal upper GI haemorrhage*
- *Consider elective intubation* to protect the airway if there is a severe uncontrolled bleed, severe encephalopathy, or evidence of aspiration
- *Urgent endoscopy* with variceal banding or sclerotherapy
- *Consider vasopressin infusion* +/– nitroglycerine, or somatostatin infusion
- A *Sengstaken–Blakemore tube* may be temporarily used to control the bleeding until definitive therapy is arranged (which may require transfer to a liver unit for transjugular intrahepatic porto-systemic shunt (TIPSS)[88] insertion or surgery).

Management of gastric varices

These are managed by endoscopic methods, surgery, or radiological intervention. There is no role at present for pharmacological management.

Prognosis

Mortality is approximately 50% for the first episode of variceal bleeding. The severity of cirrhosis (determined by the Child–Pugh classification, *see* Table 7.8) is the best prognostic predictor.

---

87 Cirrhosis is the most common cause of oesophageal varices.
88 Transjugular intrahepatic porto-systemic stent shunt insertion. This may be superior to endoscopic therapy alone.

Table 7.8   Child–Pugh score of assessing severity of cirrhosis

Score	1	2	3
Encephalopathy (grade)	0	I/II	III/IV
Ascites	Absent	Mild/moderate	Severe
Bilirubin (µmol/l)	<34	34–51	>51
Albumin (g/l)	>35	28–35	<28
INR	<1.3	1.3–1.5	>1.5

Score:
<7 (Grade A) = low risk of death
7–9 (Grade B) = moderate risk of death
10–15 (Grade C) = high risk of death.

Lower gastrointestinal haemorrhage

Incidence

Accounts for approximately one-fifth of all acute gastrointestinal bleeds.

Risk factors

Age (most common in elderly), risks associated with cause, e.g. diet and diverticular disease.

Causes

The causes of lower gastrointestinal haemorrhage include:

- *diverticular disease**
- *angiodysplasia**
- *anal pathology* – anal fissure, haemorrhoids
- *ischaemic colitis*
- *inflammatory bowel disease*
- *infective diarrhoea*
- *colonic malignancy/polyps*
- *Meckel's diverticulum.***

*Most common causes of significant lower gastrointestinal haemorrhage in adults.
**Most common cause in children.

Diverticular bleeding

Although diverticulae are more common in the sigmoid colon, bleeding often arises from diverticulae in the right colon.[89] They develop at the site where nutrient vessels penetrate the wall of the colon. Bleeding occurs when these vessels rupture into a diverticulum. Diverticular bleeding will resolve spontaneously in 90% of cases.

---

89 Longstreth GF (1997) Epidemiology and outcome of patients hospitalized with acute lower gastrointestinal hemorrhage: a population-based study. *Am J Gastroenterol* **92**: 419–24.

Angiodyplasia

This is a vascular malformation of intestinal vessels and can occur in any part of the colon but is most common on the right side.[90] There is an association with cardiac valvular abnormalities (particularly aortic stenosis). Angiodyplastic bleeding will resolve spontaneously in 80% of cases.

Anal pathology

Bleeding from haemorrhoids or from an anal fissure is usually fresh and noticed on toilet paper after wiping. However in some cases haemorrhoidal bleeding can be profuse.

Inflammatory bowel disease

See 'Emergencies in inflammatory bowel disease', page 145.

Infective diarrhoea

Common causative organisms in the UK include *Shigella, Campylobacter, Salmonella* and *E. coli.*

Colonic malignancy

This is an infrequent but important cause of lower GI haemorrhage.[91]

Ischaemic colitis

See 'Acute intestinal ischaemia', page 212.

---

90 Hochter W, Weingart J, Kuhner W *et al.* (1985) Angiodysplasia in the colon and rectum. Endoscopic morphology, localisation and frequency. *Endoscopy* **17**: 182–5.
91 Overt bleeding due to colorectal malignancy is most often caused by rectosigmoid lesions.

Symptoms

Patients present with *rectal bleeding*.[92] Other symptoms depend on the cause:

- *abdominal pain* (infective diarrhoea, colitis, diverticular disease)
- preceding *change in bowel habit* (colitis, malignancy)
- *weight loss* (malignancy)
- *anal pain* (anal pathology).

Signs

These depend on the cause and the amount of bleeding and may include:

- *anaemia*
- *shock*: due to hypovolaemia
- *abdominal tenderness*: e.g. diverticular bleeding
- *anal tenderness*: e.g. anal fissure
- *blood on DRE*
- *rectal mass on DRE*: rectal polyp, malignancy.

Investigations

- *Blood tests*: as for upper gastrointestinal bleeding – FBC, U&Es, LFTs, clotting, G&S; cross-match in severe bleeds
- *AXR*: consider if colitis may be the underlying cause
- *Rigid sigmoidoscopy* may identify the cause.

Treatment

- *Stratify the patient based on the severity of haemorrhage.*
- If there has been a *minor* bleed, allow oral fluids and admit for observation.
- If there has been a *significant* bleed (+/– haemodynamic instability):
  - *NBM*
  - *insert two large-bore cannulas*
  - *fluid resuscitation*. Transfuse if the patient is clinically shocked, or if Hb <10 g/dl and the patient is still actively bleeding
  - *urinary catheter* with *accurate fluid balance*
  - *correct clotting* if deranged
  - *consider OGD* if there is haemodynamic instability to exclude an upper GI cause

---

92 The colour of the blood and its association with stool may indicate the site of bleeding. Bright red blood noticed on the paper after wiping, or dribbling into the pan after defaecation, suggests an anorectal cause. Dark blood and clots mixed in with stool suggest that bleeding is occurring more proximally in the colon.

- *if the OGD is negative consider angiography[93]/radionuclide red cell scan[94]*
- *lower gastrointestinal bleeds are usually self-limiting.* Patients should have daily FBC and an accurate stool chart. Flexible sigmoidoscopy should be performed whilst as an inpatient, to identify the source of bleeding and, if possible, any treatment, e.g. polypectomy.

Indications for surgery

- *Hypotension despite adequate resuscitation*
- *Continued bleeding* (>6 units blood transfused) and *failure or unavailability of non-operative management* (e.g. angiography).

Surgery usually involves segmental excision of the affected segment of colon.[95]

---

93 Can localise bleeding if rate is >1 ml/min. The procedure allows therapeutic intervention (e.g. embolisation of the bleeding vessel).
94 Can localise bleeding when the rate is 0.5 ml/min but does not allow therapeutic intervention.
95 Subtotal colectomy may be necessary if the source of bleeding is unknown. In this situation an on-table angiogram may be extremely helpful in identifying where the bleeding is arising from.

Clostridium difficile diarrhoea and pseudomembranous colitis

C. difficile is a Gram-positive anaerobic bacillus which is transmitted via the faecal–oral route. This is an important noscomial pathogen that can cause diarrhoea in hospital patients.

Risk of colonisation increases with:

- length of hospital stay
- antibiotic treatment: alters the normal colonic flora
- age
- recent gastrointestinal surgery
- steroid treatment.

A proportion of those colonised will develop symptoms.

Symptoms

Lower abdominal pain, diarrhoea, fever.

Diagnosis

- *WCC + CRP elevated*
- *Detection of C. difficile exotoxin* in the stool.[96]

Treatment

- *Fluid resuscitation* and *correction of electrolyte abnormalities*
- *Stop exisiting antibiotic treatment* if possible
- *Oral metronidazole* (400 mg tds) or *oral vancomycin* (125 mg qds) for 14 days.

Pseudomembranous colitis

This occurs in severe *C. difficile* infection. Yellowish mucosal plaques seen at sigmoidoscopy are diagnostic. Symptoms are similar to the above but can include *bloody diarrhoea, abdominal distension and systemic sepsis.*

Treatment

As above. There is a risk of *toxic megacolon* which may require surgery.

---

96 This is a highly specific test. Sensitivity is between 80% and 90%. Results will usually take 48 h after the sample is taken (cytotoxin assay).

Stomas

These are created when part of the gastrointestinal tract is exteriorised to the skin. Stomas can be urostomies (usually via an ileal conduit), ileostomies or colostomies.[97] They may be temporary or permanent and fashioned as an end or loop stoma.

If a patient is likely to require a stoma during surgery, seek advice from a stoma nurse for pre-operative siting and counselling.

High-output stomas, particularly ileostomies, may result in electrolyte disturbances and dehydration. Patients may need admission for fluid resuscitation and correction of electrolytes. Strategies to reduce stoma output (e.g. loperamide) may be necessary.

Local complications can occur in up to 50–60% of cases.

Risk factors for local stoma complications

- Obesity
- Poor surgical technique
- No pre-operative siting
- Diabetes mellitus
- Smoking
- Underlying disease process such as Crohn's disease.

Skin problems

Skin problems are more common with ileostomies (due to the irritant nature of effluent). Involve the stoma nurse early. Topical steroids may have a role in treatment. Occasionally the stoma needs to be revised.

Stomal prolapse

Prolapse occurs when redundant bowel invades the stoma, caused by pressure within the abdominal cavity. It is often seen in the distal limb of a loop stoma. Transverse colostomies are especially prone to prolapse. Attempt gentle manual reduction. Osmotic therapy (e.g. finely granulated sugar sprinkled onto the mucosa) may aid reduction of the prolapse. Some patients may need refashioning or resiting of the stoma.

---

97 Ileostomies are normally found on the right side and have a mucosal spout. Colostomies are normally on the left and flush with the skin.

Stomal retraction

The risk of this is highest in obese patients. It may cause skin irritation, abdominal wall infection/abscess or peritonitis depending on the degree of retraction. A retracted stoma should therefore be revised early.

Parastomal hernia

Hernias occur in about 5% of ileostomies and up to 10% of colostomies. Small reducible hernias may be managed with a stoma belt. Complications are as for any other type of hernia. Strangulation requires immediate surgery. Surgery may involve local repair through a peristomal incision or relocation of the stoma.[98]

Bowel obstruction caused by stomal stenosis

This is relatively uncommon and may necessitate resection with repositioning of the stoma.

---

98 Relocation may be superior to fascial repair, but for recurrent parastomal hernias mesh repair may be the best solution. *See* Rubin MS, Schoetz DJ Jr and Matthews JB (1994) Parastomal hernia. Is stoma relocation superior to fascial repair? *Arch Surg* **129**: 413–18.

Abdominal compartment syndrome

Definition

An acute increase in intra-abdominal pressure[99] associated with the following physiological consequences:

- *increased cardiac afterload* and therefore reduced cardiac output
- *reduced lung compliance* and therefore reduced gas exchange
- *increased renal arterial resistance* causing oliguria/anuria
- *reduced splanchnic perfusion* leading to increased translocation of bacteria across the gut mucosa and sepsis
- *cognitive impairment* by increasing intracranial pressure.

Causes

- *Post-operative haemorrhage*
- *Ruptured AAA*
- *Abdominal trauma*
- *Bowel obstruction*
- *Ascites.*

Treatment

- *Transfer the patient to HDU/ITU*
- *Treat any reversible causes*
- *Surgical decompression* may have a role.

---

99 Intra-abdominal pressure is best recorded by measuring the intravesical pressure. Instill 50 ml of water into the bladder and then pass a catheter into the bladder attached to a manometer. Rough readings can be obtained by measuring the height of a column of urine with the urinary catheter tubing held above the level of the patient. Normal intra-abdominal pressure is less than 10 cm H_2O. A diagnosis of abdominal compartment syndrome requires a pressure of more than 25 cm H_2O.

Swallowed foreign body

Most foreign bodies pass harmlessly through the gut.

History

Ask about:

- when the foreign body was ingested
- what was swallowed
- sensation of the foreign body (e.g. sticking)
- dysphagia or drooling
- shortness of breath/stridor: the foreign body may have entered into the airway
- vomiting/abdominal pain: suggestive of bowel obstruction or perforation
- haematemesis or PR bleeding.

Examination

- *Look inside the oropharynx* for evidence of the foreign body
- *Chest signs*: reduced air entry, breath sounds or wheeze (inhaled foreign body)
- *Abdominal signs*: tenderness, distension and abnormal bowel sounds (foreign body causing obstruction/perforation).

Investigations

This will depend on the likely location of the foreign body.

- *Plain X-rays*: throat/chest/abdomen
- *Barium swallow*: if a radiolucent foreign body is likely to be in the oesophagus.

Management

- *Manage the airway* (call an anaesthetist if the airway is compromised)
- Call an *ear, nose and throat (ENT)* specialist if the foreign body is impacted in the *throat*

- A foreign body stuck in the *oesophagus*[100] should be removed *endoscopically*. However blunt foreign bodies (except button batteries) that are well tolerated may be observed for 24 h
- If a blunt foreign body reaches the *stomach* and the patient is asymptomatic it will usually *pass through the gut*[101]
- *Sharp foreign bodies* that reach the *stomach* should be removed *endoscopically*
- *Button batteries* that reach the *stomach* should probably be *removed*, as they may erode through the bowel wall
- If a *sharp foreign body* or *button battery* has passed *beyond the stomach*, the patient should be *admitted* and *observed* with *regular imaging*.

Indications for laparotomy

- *Failure to remove a sharp foreign body endoscopically*
- *Obstruction*
- *Signs of peritonitis* suggestive of perforation
- *Catastrophic bleed*
- *Failure of a button battery to progress through the gut in a 24 h period.*

Foreign body in the rectum

This may present late. Consider perforation if abdominal pain is a feature. Removal may require a GA. Removal can usually be achieved via a trans-anal approach. However laparotomy is occasionally necessary (consent the patient for this and the possibility of a stoma).

---

100 Foregn bodies that get 'stuck' in the oesophagus usually do so at the level of the cricopharyngeus, but also at the mid-oesophagus and at the level of the lower oesophageal sphincter.
101 The narrowest part of the alimentary tract is at the level of cricopharyngeus in the throat. Therefore most items that pass the throat will pass through the rest of the gut.

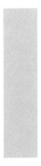

Chapter 8

Anorectal emergencies

Anorectal sepsis

Anorectal sepsis is a common condition accounting for a large proportion of acute surgical admissions. It occurs most frequently in the third and fourth decades, and is more common in males (3:1).

A significant number of patients develop chronic sepsis and fistula formation. Rarely, complications such as necrotising fasciitis can arise from an anorectal abscess.

Primary anorectal abscess

Skin-related abscesses

These arise from infection of apocrine glands or hair follicles surrounding the anal margin. Culture of organisms usually generates skin flora. They are not commonly associated with fistula formation.

Anal gland infections

Eisenhammer (1956) and Parks (1961) proposed the 'cryptoglandular theory' of anorectal sepsis, and anal gland infection is now accepted as the commonest source of anorectal sepsis. The anal glands are situated between the internal and external sphincter at the level of the dentate line, and communicate with the mucosa and submucosa via ducts arising from the anal valves. Infection of the anal gland can result in chronic abscess formation in the intersphincteric space. This infection may spread in a number of directions (*see* Figure 8.1):

- downwards in the intersphincteric space resulting in a *perianal abscess* (commonest)
- penetration across the external sphincter resulting in an *ischiorectal abscess* which occasionally extends upwards to form a *supralevator abscess*
- upwards in the intersphincteric space resulting in a high *intersphincteric abscess* or *supralevator abscess.*

Circumferential spread (*see* Figure 8.2) in the ischiorectal, or more rarely perianal or supralevator planes results in a horseshoe abscess.

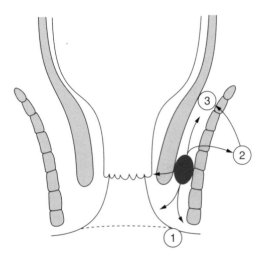

Figure 8.1 Spread of infection: 1, perianal abscess; 2, ischiorectal abscess; 3, supralevator abscess.

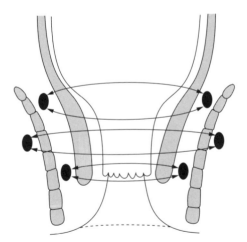

Figure 8.2 Circumferential spread of infection.

Secondary anorectal abscess

Secondary anorectal abscesses are associated with underlying disease:

- *Crohn's disease*
- *malignancy*
- *immunosuppression*: e.g. diabetes, leukaemia, AIDS or steroid treatment
- *atypical infection*: TB, actinomycosis, amoebiasis, schistosomiasis and fungal
- *other anal pathology*
- *iatrogenic*: e.g. sclerotherapy, banding or excision of haemorrhoids.

Symptoms

Gradual onset of *perianal pain, swelling* and *fever*. Pain may be exarcerbated by defaecation.

Signs

Pyrexia, red tender swelling of the perianal skin.

Treatment

- *Admit*
- *NBM*
- *Analgesia*
- *Surgical drainage*: EUA + incision and drainage under GA.

There is a risk of recurrence and of fistula formation.

Prolapsed strangulated haemorrhoids

Haemorrhoids are common and occur when the normal 'vascular cushions' of the anal canal become enlarged. They may present acutely with strangulation.

Pathogenesis of strangulation

As haemorrhoids enlarge they protrude through the anus. The anus acts as a constricting agent causing vascular compromise with resulting infarction and thrombosis of the haemorrhoid.

Symptoms

Severe anal *pain* with a *swelling* protruding through the anus.

Signs

Tender dark red or purple swelling protruding through the anal canal (usually in the 3, 7 or 11 o'clock positions).[1]

Treatment

There are two ways of treating strangulated haemorrhoids:

- symptomatic treatment with *ice packs, laxatives/stool softeners* and *analgesia*. The majority of cases settle within 10 days. Subsequent haemorrhoidectomy is advised to prevent recurrence
- if the symptoms are severe then there is a case for *emergency haemorrhoidectomy*.

---

1   A thrombosed pile must be differentiated from a rectal prolapse. Prolapses are usually paler in appearance, have concentric mucosal rings, and a double layer on bimanual palpation.

Thrombosed perianal varix (perianal haematoma)

Pathogenesis

Uncertain. There is some evidence that sudden tearing of the anal margin following an episode of diarrhoea or constipation precipitates thrombosis of a venous saccule in the perianal submucosal venous plexus.

Symptoms

Severe *anal pain* with a *perianal swelling*, which usually develops over 24–48 h. Patients may experience *difficulty passing stool*.

Signs

Blue smooth tender lump lying subcutaneously at the anal margin.

Treatment

Treat symptoms with *ice packs* and *topical analgesia*. This is usually sufficient as the condition is self-limiting. If pain is severe consider evacuation of the haematoma under LA.

Rectal prolapse

Risk factors

Increasing age (5th decade upwards), female (85% cases), any cause of pelvic floor weakness. Constipation may be an independent risk factor.

Pathogenesis

Uncertain. Most patients with full-thickness rectal prolapse have a weak atonic anal sphincter and/or weak pelvic floor.

Symptoms

Painless swelling protruding from the anus after defaecation or during any episode of raised intra-abdominal pressure (e.g. coughing). There is usually a background of incontinence of faeces and flatus, with urgency and episodes of soiling. A tendency to constipation is common.

Signs

- *Non-tender red swelling* protruding through anal canal with visible folds of mucosa
- Rarely the prolapse becomes *gangrenous* due to vascular compromise.

Treatment

Manual reduction of the prolapse. Patients should have a sigmoidoscopy to exclude additional rectal pathology. *Dietary modification* and *laxatives* may help. The patient will need outpatient assessment with a view to surgical treatment. Surgery is only indicated acutely if there has been infarction of the prolapse.

Pilonidal abscess

Risk factors

Young adult, male, generous covering of body hair.

Pathogenesis

Abscess formation within the subcutaneous tissue of the natal cleft follows infection of a pilonidal sinus. There is ongoing debate about whether pilonidal sinuses are a congenital or acquired condition. Current evidence favours an acquired cause. It is thought the sinus forms when hair (either rooted locally or from elsewhere) penetrates the skin of the natal cleft. Movement of the buttocks propels the hair deeper into the skin. Barbs on the hair prevent expulsion.

Symptoms

Pain and *swelling* in the natal cleft region. Patients may be *systemically unwell with fever*.

Signs

- *Red hot swelling* in the natal cleft
- Presence of *midline pit(s)*
- There may be *inguinal lymphadenopathy*
- The patient may be unwell with signs of *systemic sepsis*.

Treatment

- *Admit*
- *NBM*
- *Analgesia*
- *Surgery*: the abscess should be *incised and drained* under GA
- If the patient has signs of systemic sepsis and there is likely to be a significant delay before surgical drainage *broad-spectrum intravenous antibiotics should be considered*.

Chapter 9

Vascular emergencies

Deep venous thrombosis

A thrombosis is a solid mass formed from blood constituents that develops within flowing blood.[1]

Incidence

1 in 1000.

Site of origin

The most frequent site is in the deep veins of the calf. The less common popliteal, femoral, or ilio-femoral thrombi[2] (proximal DVT) are more serious due to the much higher risk of pulmonary embolism. However, one-fifth of untreated newly developing calf vein thrombi extend proximally. DVTs can also occur in upper limbs in association with trauma or thoracic inlet syndrome.

Risk factors

- *Increasing age*
- *Pregnancy*
- *Malignancy*
- *Previous history of DVT*
- *Varicose veins*
- *Obesity*
- *Immobility*
- *Protein C/protein S deficiency.*

Symptoms

- *Swollen limb*
- *Calf pain*
- *Fever.*

---

1 A *clot* in contrast is a solid mass formed from the constituents of blood in stationary blood.

2 Ileofemoral DVT may present with *phlegmasia alba dolens* (PAD) or *phlegmasia cerulea dolens* (PCD): the former is a swollen white leg with blanching (caused by subcutaneous oedema); the latter is a blue leg with cyanosis due to propagation of venous thrombus at the microcapillary level and secondary ischaemia (venous gangrene may result). Underlying malignant disease is usually responsible for PCD. Prognosis is poor.

DVT may be *asymptomatic* and present with clinical features of pulmonary embolism.

Signs

- *Pyrexia* (low grade)
- *Calf tenderness*
- *Distension of the superficial veins*
- *Increased limb girth.*

Differential diagnosis of DVT

- *Cellulitis*
- *Superficial thrombophlebitis*
- *Ruptured Baker's cyst*
- *Haematoma in muscle*
- *Muscle tear or strain*
- *Dependent oedema*
- *Post-thrombotic syndrome*
- *Lymphatic obstruction*
- *Arthritis*
- *Heart failure, cirrhosis, nephrotic syndrome*
- *External compression of major veins* (e.g. by foetus, cancer)
- *Arterio-venous fistula.*

Investigations

- *D-Dimer blood test*: highly sensitive. However levels may be elevated in post-operative patients irrespective of whether a DVT is present
- *Duplex ultrasound*: less accurate than *venography* in diagnosing *calf thrombosis* (but non-invasive). If the duplex is normal but symptoms support the diagnosis the patient should be rescanned after one week
- *Venography* is the gold standard and should be performed when the diagnosis is still uncertain after non-invasive testing.[3]

Patients who have a proven DVT should be screened for factor V Leiden deficiency, and protein C and S deficiencies.

---

3   Kearon C, Julian JA, Newman TE and Ginsberg JS (1998) Noninvasive diagnosis of deep venous thrombosis. *Ann Intern Med* **128**: 663–77.

Treatment

Usually managed by the physicians. Surgical management may be appropriate in some circumstances.

- *Graduated compression stockings*
- *Low-molecular-weight heparin (LMWH):*[4] prevents propagation of established thrombus and the development of pulmonary embolism
- *Warfarin:* maintenance anticoagulation with oral anticoagulants (unless pregnant) following initial heparinisation. Optimal target INR = 2.5; duration of treatment should be 3 months after the first episode of DVT
- *Thrombolysis:* may be indicated for patients with severe DVT causing critical limb ischaemia, or for those with massive pulmonary embolism (PE)
- *Surgery:* venous thrombectomy for proximal DVT may reduce venous reflux and post-thrombotic sequelae[5]
- *Inferior vena caval filter:* occasionally used when anticoagulation is contra-indicated or when adequate anticoagulation fails to prevent recurrent embolism.

Complications of DVT

- *Pulmonary embolism (PE):* 10% incidence of symptomatic PE in untreated proximal DVT
- *Critical limb ischaemia:* severe DVT can result in extremely high venous pressures and impairment of arterial blood flow
- *Recurrent DVTs:* risk of recurrent venous thromboembolism is reduced if anticoagulated; >20% of DVTs recur within 5 years
- *Post-thrombotic syndrome* (chronic venous insufficiency with subsequent venous ulceration): complicates 50–75% of DVTs. Compression stockings may significantly reduce the risk.[6]

---

4 LMWH has the advantage of simpler dose titration, once-daily subcutaneous administration, no need for routine laboratory monitoring, and cost-effectiveness compared to unfractionated heparin. *See* Gould MK, Dembitzer AD, Doyle R *et al.* (1999) Low-molecular-weight heparins compared with unfractionated heparin for treatment of acute deep venous thrombosis. *Ann Intern Med* **130**: 800–9.

5 Plate G, Eklof B, Norgren L *et al.* (1997) Venous thrombectomy for iliofemoral vein thrombosis – 10-year results of a prospective randomised study. *Eur J Vasc Endovasc Surg* **14**: 367–74.

6 Brandjes DP, Buller HR, Heijboer H *et al.* (1997) Randomised trial of effect of compression stockings in patients with symptomatic proximal-vein thrombosis. *The Lancet* **349**: 759–62.

Lower limb ulceration

When examining ulcers, assess:

- shape
- size
- position
- colour
- temperature
- tenderness
- base of ulcer
- edge of ulcer
- depth
- any associated lymphadenopathy.

Varicose/venous ulcers

Chronic venous insufficiency due to impairment of venous return results in increased venous pressure and oedema. This leads to *venous eczema* and *lipodermatosclerosis* (fibrosis and the deposition of haemosiderin). Excess proteolytic activity and fibrinolysis together with minor trauma lead to ulceration. Typical features of venous ulcers are shown in Table 9.1.

Ulcers may be of mixed aetiology and therefore arterial disease needs to be excluded.

Investigations

- *Exclude arterial disease* (*see* investigations for arterial ulcers, page 197)
- *Exclude infection:*[7] take swabs, X-ray to exclude osteomyelitis
- *Venous duplex.*

Treatment

- *Elevate the limb* in order to reduce oedema
- *Four-layer graduated compression therapy* using elastic bandaging (pressure of 40 mmHg at ankle). Be cautious when applying to patients with cardiac failure, as the increased venous return may have adverse consequences

---

7 Ulcers are most commonly infected by group A *Streptococci* and *Staphylococcus aureus*, although in diabetic or immunocompromised patients Gram-negative bacilli may be responsible. Treat empirically with penicillin + flucloxacillin while awaiting culture results.

Table 9.1   Characteristics and treatment of four major types of ulceration

Type of ulceration	Characteristics	Treatment
Venous	F > M, gaiter area, shallow, irregular, can be painful, preceding history of venous disease, lipodermatosclerosis, venous eczema, oedema	Elevation to reduce oedema Compression (typically four-layer) Treat infection Debridement +/– skin graft
Arterial	History of arterial disease (claudication and rest pain) Risk factors (smoking, diabetes, cardiac disease, hypertension, high cholesterol, family history) Ulcers are over bony areas in feet, deep, circumscribed and not irregular, necrotic, +/– absent pulses	Address risk factors Improve arterial supply, either through angioplasty or bypass Amputation
Neuropathic (diabetic)	Plantar aspect of foot Poorly controlled diabetes Foot may be deformed (Charcot's joint) Abnormal neurological findings	Podiatry Control of diabetes Improve arterial supply if macrovascular disease
Pressure ulcers	Sacrum or heel Patient invariably disabled or bed-bound Prolonged pressure leads to tissue necrosis	Release pressure over affected area (podiatry if foot ulcer) Nutrition Treat infection Debridement

- *Intermittent pneumatic compression* may be a useful adjunct to elastic bandaging
- *Aspirin* may be beneficial.[8]

---

8   Layton AM, Ibbotson SH, Davies JA *et al.* (1994) Randomised trial of oral aspirin for chronic venous leg ulcers. *The Lancet* **344**: 164–5.

Surgical options

Surgery is probably only of benefit in ulcers that fail to respond to conservative therapy. Consider:

● *venous surgery*: useful in those with superficial venous incompetence. Subfascial endoscopic perforator surgery (SEPS) may also have a role
● *surgical debridement*: removal of necrotic tissue
● *biopsy*: especially in ulcers with raised edges (to exclude malignancy[9])
● *skin grafting*: can be split-skin or pinch grafting under local anaesthetic.

Arterial ulcers

Features of arterial ulcers are shown in Table 9.1.

Investigations

● *Exclude infection*: take swabs, X-ray to exclude osteomyelitis
● *Ankle brachial pressure indices* (ABPIs)[10]
● *Arterial duplex scan*
● *Consider angiography/magnetic resonance angiography* (MRA).

Treatment

● *Control of risk factors* (stop smoking, control hypertension, diabetes and cholesterol)
● *Angioplasty*
● *Consider bypass surgery.*

Neuropathic ulcers

These are usually seen in patients with *diabetic neuropathy*. Typical features are shown in Table 9.1.

Treatment

● *Good diabetic control*
● *Control of other risk factors*

---

9 Squamous cell carcinoma developing in long-standing ulcer (Marjolin's ulcer).
10 ABPI < 0.9 indicates arterial insufficiency (in non-diabetics). An ulcer with both arterial and venous components in the presence of an ABPI < 0.5 will not heal without improvement of arterial inflow.

- *Good foot care.* Refer to podiatry
- *Treat infection aggressively*
- *Early debridement.*

Pressure ulcers

These tend to occur in *debilitated individuals* or those who are *paralysed.* Sacral and heel sores occur commonly on geriatric wards. It is important to *ensure good nutrition. Surgical debridement* +/– plastic surgery may be appropriate.

Acute lower limb ischaemia

A sudden decrease in limb perfusion that results in symptoms and signs of ischaemia.

Causes

- *Thrombosis:*[11] the commonest cause. Usually due to rupture of an athero-sclerotic plaque and platelet aggregation. Thrombosis can also occur after limb surgery and in popliteal aneurysms
- *Embolism:* atrial fibrillation (AF) or mural thrombus after an MI are the commonest causes. Emboli can also arise from the aorta, particularly if the patient has an AAA,[12] or from cardiac valves (ask about previous rheumatic fever and risk factors for infective endocarditis)
- *Trauma: see* 'Vascular trauma', page 70.

Differential diagnosis

Consider the following other diagnoses which may mimic acute limb ischaemia:

- *cardiac failure* in a patient who already has diseased limb vessels
- *ileofemoral DVT.*

Features of acute ischaemia

The *Six 'P's*:

- pain
- pallor
- paralysis
- paraesthesia
- pulselessness
- perishingly cold leg.

Paralysis is a *late symptom* that occurs when muscle infarction has already begun. *Paraesthesia* in contrast is an *early symptom*.

---

11 Risk factors for atherosclerosis are hypertension, diabetes, smoking, family history and high cholesterol.
12 Emboli from vessels are likely to be multiple and can lodge in very distal vessels.

Ask about *symptoms of intermittent claudication.*[13] A preceding history of claudication suggests a thrombotic rather than embolic aetiology.

Examination

- *Examine the cardiovascular system*: AF, heart murmur
- *Exclude AAA.*

Next assess the limbs and compare:

- colour[14]
- temperature
- scars indicating previous vascular surgery
- signs of chronic ischaemia (e.g. hair loss, ulceration)
- sensation + power
- pulses (*see* Box 9.1). A handheld Doppler probe may be useful for this
- capillary refill.

Box 9.1   Pulses in the lower limb

- *Femoral pulse*: at the mid-inguinal point (mid-way between the pubic symphysis and the anterior superior iliac spine)
- *Popliteal pulse*:[15] flex the knee 45°. The popliteal pulse is felt in the centre of the popliteal fossa
- *Posterior tibial pulse*: felt behind the medial malleolus
- *Dorsalis pedis pulse*: felt between the first and second metatarsal bones (lateral to the extensor hallucis longus tendon).

---

13 This is muscle pain due to ischaemia. It characteristically occurs in the calf (and sometimes the thigh and buttocks) on exercise, and is relieved by rest. *Neurogenic claudication* in contrast is associated with back pain and pain on prolonged standing, and is relieved by leaning forward.

14 The colour of the affected limb may offer a clue as to the duration of ischaemia. In the initial few hours the limb becomes pale and white. Subsequently there is a mottled appearance with blanching on pressure. After 12 h, there is irreversible ischaemia, and the limb has fixed mottling with no blanching. In patients who have pre-existing vascular disease (and therefore the presence of collaterals), it is likely that the limb may remain in the initial stages for some time, with very slow progression to irreversible ischaemia.

15 Remember to look for a popliteal aneurysm which may be the source of emboli.

Investigations

The following should be performed.

- *FBC*: Hb and platelets may be elevated if there is hypercoagulability
- *U&Es*: electrolytes + renal function
- *Check clotting*
- *G&S*
- *ECG*
- Consider *duplex scan/angiogram* (*see* 'Treatment' below).

Treatment

- *Admit*
- *Analgesia*
- *Resuscitation* (i.v. fluids, control AF)
- *Oxygen*
- *Raise the head of the bed*
- *Start heparin infusion*
- *Urgent surgical embolectomy*: an embolic cause is likely if symptoms are of sudden onset and there is no pre-existing claudication. The patient should also have a full set of contralateral pulses and the presence of a potential source of emboli (e.g. AF). If embolectomy is unsuccessful then the patient should have an on-table angiogram with reconstruction thereafter
- *Urgent angiogram +/– thrombolysis*: angiography may be appropriate when the cause is uncertain. Thrombolysis can be delivered locally via the arteriography catheter[16]
- *Surgical revascularisation*: consider if thrombolysis[17] fails
- In patients with significant co-morbidity or a non-salvageable limb, *palliative measures* may be appropriate.

---

16 Thrombolysis is fraught with complications. The patient should be warned of the possibility of haemorrhage (1 in 10) and risks of stroke. The contraindications to initial thrombolytic therapy include active bleeding, pregnancy, recent stroke, recent surgery, coagulopathy, presence of aneurysm and previous GI bleeding. Reports of success of thrombolysis are variable in the literature. Limb salvage occurs in about 70% of patients. Thrombolysis is less successful in those patients who are older, are diabetic, and who have a vein graft occlusion. Furthermore if the patient has diffuse disease in the affected limb, thrombolysis is less likely to succeed.

17 Even if thrombolysis is effective, the patient will probably need definitive treatment (angioplasty, stent insertion or surgical bypass) subsequently. *See* Ouriel K and Veith FJ (1998) Acute lower limb ischemia: determinants of outcome. *Surgery* **124**: 336–41.

Determinants of outcome

The following variables have been shown to be predictive of amputation-free survival:[18]

- white race
- younger age
- absence of central nervous disease, malignancy, cardiac failure
- absence of skin colour changes
- absence of pain at rest.

18 Ouriel K and Veith FJ (1998) Acute lower limb ischaemia: determinants of outcome. *Surgery* **124**: 336–41.

Acute upper limb ischaemia

This is less common than lower limb ischaemia, and is usually due to thrombo-embolism or trauma.

Incidence

2 per 100 000. F = M.

Causes

Embolism is the most common cause. Sources of emboli include:

- *the heart*: AF, mural thrombus, valvular disease
- *the aortic arch*
- *subclavian aneurysm* (which may be associated with a cervical rib).

In at least one in 10 patients, a source of embolism is never found.

Thrombosis can also occur, but is rarer and often associated with malignancy. Other rarer causes include arterial dissection, vibration vasospasm and connective tissue disease.[19]

Management

The management of upper limb ischaemia is essentially *similar to lower limb ischaemia*. However there are a few additional important points:

- *history*: ask about *hand dominance* and *occupation*
- *examination*: assess the *supraclavicular fossa* to look for an aneurysm or cervical rib
- *investigations*: *blood tests* (as for lower limb ischaemia); *CXR* may demonstrate the cause
- *treatment*: as emboli are a more common cause in the upper limb, urgent *brachial embolectomy* should be undertaken in most patients.[20]

---

19 Raynaud's phenomenon is a possible differential diagnosis. Typically there is a characteristic triphasic colour change in the fingers: white (vasospasm), blue (cyanosis) and then red (reperfusion). Raynaud's syndrome may be a secondary feature of other disease (e.g. connective tissue disorders).

20 Conservative management should be considered for those who present with mild symptoms (i.e. no paralysis and minimal pain), or for those with significant co-morbidity. The latter may preclude surgery even under local anaesthetic. Limb loss is rare although patients may lose full function.

Digital infarcts

These are caused by small emboli. Consider *angiography* (+/– angioplasty of any proximal stenosis). *Iloprost infusion* may be useful in improving digital microcirculation.

Aortic dissection

This is caused by blood breaking through the intima and establishing a false passage in the media of the vessel wall. Aetiological factors include Marfan's (especially type 2 dissection), hypertension, cystic medial necrosis, infection and trauma.

Aortic dissection is classified into three types (DeBakey classification):

- *type 1*: affects both the ascending and descending aorta
- *type 2*: affects the ascending aorta alone
- *type 3*: affects the aorta distal to the left subclavian artery.

Symptoms and signs

These depend on the location of the dissection and whether it tracks proximally or distally:

- classically a *tearing chest pain* radiating to the back
- *shock*
- *disparate blood pressures* between *upper limbs*
- if the dissection tracks proximally it may give rise to a *stroke, upper limb ischaemia, MI, aortic regurgitation* (new aortic diastolic heart murmur) or *cardiac tamponade*
- if the dissection tracks distally it can cause *renal failure* or *disruption of lower limb arterial* inflow.[21]

Investigations

The following should be performed:

- *blood tests*: FBC, U&Es, clotting, cross-match blood
- *ECG*
- *CXR* (widened mediastinum, loss of aortic knob, pleural effusion)
- *CT* will allow better definition of the dissection
- consider *trans-oesophageal echo (TOE)*.

---

21 These additional symptoms of aortic dissection relating to branch occlusion occur in 10–20% of patients.

Treatment

- *Admit*
- *Resuscitate*
- *Analgesia*
- All *proximal dissections* (type 1 and type 2) should be treated *surgically*. Discuss with the *Cardiothoracic* department
- *Type 3 dissections* should be managed *medically*. This involves blood pressure control (lowered to 100–110 mmHg systolic). Endovascular management may be an option, and involves the insertion of a stent-graft across the primary tear. Surgery is reserved for those dissections that rupture.

Ruptured abdominal aortic aneurysm (AAA)

Aneurysms

An aneurysm is defined as a *localised abnormal dilatation of a blood vessel.*
Aneurysms can be classified as:

- *true or false*: true aneurysms incorporate all layers of the vessel wall. False
  aneurysms are surrounded by peri-vascular soft tissue
- *fusiform or saccular*
- *congenital or acquired.*

Abdominal aortic aneurysm (AAA)

An aortic diameter greater than 3 cm is aneurysmal.

Risk factors

- Males more commonly affected than females (5:1)
- Incidence increases with age (rare under the age of 60 years)
- Risk factors associated with atherosclerosis.

Pathogenesis

Loss of vessel wall elastin (possibly related to overproduction of matrix metal-
loproteinases) causing reduction in tensile strength leads to aneurysm formation. 10% of AAAs are inflammatory.

Five-year probability of rupture[22]

- 5–6 cm: 25%
- 6–7 cm: 35%
- >7 cm: 75%.

---

22 Vardulaki KA, Prevost TC, Walker NM *et al.* (1998) Growth rates and risk of
rupture of abdominal aortic aneurysms. *Br J Surg* **85**: 1674–80.

Ruptured AAA

50% die before reaching hospital and 50% of those who make it to hospital also die. Rupture may be intraperitoneal or retroperitoneal. Patients with an intra-peritoneal rupture rarely survive to reach hospital.

Symptoms and signs

These may include:

- *epigastric pain radiating to the back*
- *collapse/hypovolaemic shock*
- *tender expansile mass in the epigastrium*
- *flank ecchymosis*
- *loss of femoral pulse(s).*

Management

Speed is essential. Alert theatres and see the patient on arrival in the A&E resuscitation area.

- *Insert two large-bore cannulas*
- *Fluid resuscitation*
- *Send blood for FBC, U&Es, clotting, and cross-match 6 units blood*
- *ECG*
- *Get senior help*
- *Immediate surgery*[23] if a diagnosis of ruptured AAA has been made clinically and the patient is suitable for theatre[24]
- *CT scan* if the diagnosis is unclear and the patient is stable.

Complications of surgery

Mortality may be as high as 50%.
   Early complications include:

- bleeding
- enteric ischaemia, particularly in inferior mesenteric artery territory

---

23 Surgery involves a midline incision followed by cross-clamping the aorta proximal to the aneurysm (preferably across the infra-renal aorta). Control distally is followed by opening the sac and removing the mural thrombus. A Dacron graft is inserted (either straight or trouser), and stitched proximally and distally.

24 Consider co-existing morbidity and likely prognosis. Mortality has been shown to be 100% if there are three or more of the following: age > 76 years, creatinine > 190, Hb < 9 g/dl, ischaemic ECG changes, loss of consciousness after arrival in hospital (Hardman index). *See* Hardman DT, Fisher CM, Patel MI *et al.* (1996) Ruptured abdominal aortic aneurysms: who should be offered surgery? *J Vasc Surg* **23**: 123–9.

- multi-organ failure (related to initial shock +/– reperfusion injury)
- renal failure particularly if supra-renal clamp applied
- paraplegia due to lumbar ischaemia
- lower limb ischaemia
- trash foot (due to emboli).

Late complications include:

- sexual dysfunction
- aorto-enteric fistula
- graft infection.

Other aneurysms

Popliteal aneurysms

These are the second commonest aneurysms after AAAs. The vessel is aneurysmal if it is more than 2 cm in diameter. They are often bilateral (50% of cases).

They can:

- compress adjacent structures causing venous obstruction or neurological symptoms
- rupture (very rare)
- thrombose
- cause distal emboli.

Femoral aneurysms

These are often associated with abdominal aneurysms and usually present with *pain* (caused by local pressure), or because of thrombosis with *distal limb embolisation*. Rupture is uncommon.

Splenic artery aneurysms

These usually occur in females. Incidence rates vary from 0.02 to 0.1%. Risk factors include multiparity and portal hypertension. Rupture is most likely in the third trimester of pregnancy. They often cause *left upper quadrant pain* (especially when ruptured), and once identified (usually by CT) *aneurysectomy with splenectomy* is the treatment of choice.

Mycotic aneurysms

These develop due to infection (usually *Staphylococcus*, *Salmonella* and *Streptococcus*) in the artery wall. The commonest artery to be involved is the aorta. The patient usually presents with an *expansile mass* which may be *warm on palpation*. There is typically *fever*. CT often shows *periaortic inflammation*.

Aorto-enteric fistula

These may be primary or secondary:

- a *primary aorto-enteric fistula* usually occurs between an aneurysm and a portion of the gastrointestinal tract (usually the third part of the duodenum)
- *secondary aorto-enteric fistulae* are more common and invariably occur in a patient who has previously had an AAA repair. The fistula is usually between the proximal suture line and the distal portion of the duodenum, although it can occur with any part of the bowel.

Presentation

The patient presents with a *catastrophic GI bleed*. There may be a herald bleed prior to this which is minor and self-limiting. The time interval between the herald bleed and massive blood loss may be hours or even months.

Treatment

- It may be necessary to *proceed directly to surgery*[25]
- If the patient is *stable*, or the diagnosis is unclear, *consider an urgent upper GI endoscopy or CT.*[26]

---

25 The operation should be covered with broad-spectrum antibiotics. If the fistula involves a graft then removal of the graft becomes necessary; the aorta is oversewn and axillo-bifemoral bypass performed.
26 Signs suggestive of an aorto-enteric fistula on CT include air in the aortic wall, and thickening of the bowel wall overlying an aneurysm.

Acute intestinal ischaemia

Acute mesenteric ischaemia can affect any part of the alimentary tract but most commonly affects the small bowel or colon (otherwise known as acute ischaemic colitis).

The artery most often involved is the superior mesenteric artery (SMA) either through thrombus formation or embolus[27] from a proximal source (e.g. mural thrombus after an MI or thrombus associated with AF). Occasionally mesenteric ischaemia is caused by venous disease (associated with malignancy, sepsis, or volvulus).

Females are affected twice as often as males. Mortality is high.

Symptoms and signs

Symptoms are generally out of proportion to abdominal signs:

- sudden onset of *severe central abdominal pain*
- *vomiting*
- *blood in the stool*: suggestive of established infarction
- the *abdomen* is often *non-tender*. Signs of peritonism suggest infarcted bowel
- *bowel sounds* are usually *absent.*

Investigations

- *FBC*: elevated WCC
- *U&Es*: electrolytes + renal function
- *CRP*: elevated
- *LFTs*: may be deranged if systemic sepsis
- *Amylase*: mildly elevated
- *Check clotting*
- *G&S*
- *Arterial blood gases*: metabolic acidosis
- *ECG*
- *AXR*: may reveal a thickened bowel wall + dilatation
- *Erect CXR*: to exclude perforation.

---

27 Prognosis is worse with thrombosis. Thrombotic occlusion usually occurs at the origin of the SMA, resulting in more extensive ischaemia than embolism (which usually occurs at one of the distal branches).

Treatment

- *NBM*
- *Fluid resuscitation*
- *Analgesia*
- *Urinary catheter* with accurate fluid balance
- Consider *NG tube*
- *Broad spectrum i.v. antibiotics* (cefuroxime and metronidazole)
- *Surgery*[28]
- Consider i.v. heparin infusion post-operatively.

---

28 Surgery usually involves resection of the infarcted segment of bowel. If the bowel appears viable then it may be possible to perform a SMA embolectomy.

Chapter 10

Urological emergencies

Acute retention of urine

Incidence

Commoner in men[1] (10:1). 10% of men over the age of 60 years will experience acute retention of urine over a five-year period.

Causes

Obstructive

- Prostatic pathology (benign prostatic hyperplasia (BPH), cancer of the prostate)
- Clot retention (e.g. after surgery, frank haematuria secondary to tumour)
- Stone/tumour at the bladder neck
- Dynamic obstruction with anticholinergic drugs
- Tight phimosis
- Urethral valve (neonate) or stricture
- Bladder neck hypertrophy.

Neurological

- After pelvic or spinal surgery
- Multiple sclerosis
- Diabetic neuropathy.

Myogenic

- Overdistention (e.g. following anaesthesia or alcohol binge).

Other

- Constipation
- UTI.

---

1 A neurological cause should always be excluded in females with retention.

Symptoms

Severe lower abdominal pain associated with an *inability to void urine.* Other symptoms are associated with the underlying cause. In men the history should include questions about *lower urinary tract symptoms* (LUTS).[2]

Signs

Patient *distressed. Palpable bladder.*[3] Examination should include rectal examination (assess for constipation, sphincter tone and size of prostate) and neurological assessment.

Investigations

- *Urine dipstick* + send MSU
- *Check U&Es*: retention may cause acute renal failure
- *Consider PSA*: prostate-specific antigen.

Other investigations will depend on the likely cause.

Treatment

- *Urethral catheterisation*[4] (size 12–14 in females, 16 in males). Following renal tract decompression there may be haematuria and polyuria. Therefore *consider admission* for *observation* and *fluid management. Monitor electrolytes.* Timing of catheter removal will depend on the cause (e.g. following treatment if UTI/prostatic enlargement).

Difficult urethral catheterisation

Discuss with a Urologist. Options include:

- using a more rigid urethral catheter
- use of an introducer
- suprapubic catheterisation.

---

2 These may be *obstructive*: hesitancy, poor urine stream, terminal dribbling, or *irritative*: urgency, frequency, and nocturia.
3 In acute or chronic retention, the bladder may not be easily palpable because it becomes floppy with prolonged over-distention.
4 It may be necessary to insert a urinary catheter to relieve discomfort before carrying out a full history/examination.

Haematuria

Definition

The presence of red blood cells in urine. Haematuria can be microscopic or macroscopic.[5]

Causes of haematuria

- *Infection*: UTI, pyelonephritis, schistosomiasis, prostatitis
- *Inflammation*: glomerulonephritis, haemorrhagic cystitis (after radiotherapy)
- *Tumour*: transitional cell carcinoma (TCC)[6] (of the bladder, ureter or renal pelvis), squamous cell carcinoma (rare in the UK, commoner worldwide due to schistosomiasis), renal cell carcinoma, Wilm's tumour (children), prostate cancer
- *Other*: BPH, stones, renal papillary necrosis, strenuous exercise, trauma.

Up to 60% of patients presenting with haematuria have no identifiable cause.

History

- *Blood in the urine*: haematuria throughout the stream occurs with pathology in the bladder or higher tracts. Terminal haematuria may originate from the bladder or prostate due to compression
- *Pain* in the loin suggests stone disease or infection. Painless haematuria may suggest malignancy
- *Ask about*: LUTS, weight loss, previous symptoms from stones, presence of a bleeding disorder, anticoagulation and risk factors for neoplasia (e.g. occupation, smoking).

Signs

These can include:

- *shock*
- *anaemia*
- *palpable bladder* (if clot retention)

---

5 Macroscopic haematuria is five times more likely to be associated with a serious underlying cause than microscopic haematuria.
6 Macroscopic haematuria is the most common presentation of TCC of the urothelium.

- *palpable kidney* (if tumour, obstruction, polycystic disease)
- *enlarged prostate* on rectal examination.

Investigations

- *FBC*: Hb may be low but is usually normal
- *U&Es*: check electrolytes + renal function
- *Check clotting*
- *G&S*
- *Dip urine*[7] and send urine for *culture* and *cytology*
- *IVU* or *USS*[8]
- *Flexible cystoscopy*
- *CT/MRI* are not standard investigations but may be used in equivocal cases.

Treatment of macroscopic haematuria

- *Fluid resuscitation* if required
- Insert a *three-way urethral catheter* (size 18 to 24) for irrigation
- *Monitor electrolytes*
- *Correct coagulopathy* if present
- *Further treatment will depend on the underlying cause.*

---

7 Blood on dipstick should be confirmed by microscopy as false positives can occur, e.g. with myoglobinuria.
8 Renal parenchymal pathologies are more likely to be detected on USS, whereas IVU is better for lesions of the collecting system, e.g. TCC.

Urinary tract infection (UTI)

Definition

Bacteriuria (significant if greater than 10^5 organisms/ml) with symptoms of genitourinary inflammation at a particular site: kidney (pyelonephritis), bladder (cystitis), urethra (urethritis) or prostate (prostatitis).

UTIs occur more frequently in females due to the shorter urethra.

Risk factors

- Urinary stasis (e.g. outflow obstruction/incomplete bladder emptying, bladder diverticulae)
- Tumour
- Stone disease
- Foreign body (e.g. catheter, ureteric stent)
- Diabetes.

Pathogens

The following pathogens may cause UTI:

- *E. coli* (90% community-acquired UTIs and 50% hospital-acquired)
- *S. saprophyticus* (especially sexually active women)
- *S. aureus*
- *Proteus*
- *Klebsiella*
- *Pseudomonas* (especially in the presence of a foreign body)
- schistosomiasis is a common cause worldwide
- tuberculosis should be considered in the presence of 'sterile' pyuria[9]
- sexually transmitted organisms (e.g. *Chlamydia*).

Symptoms

These may include:

- *dysuria*
- *haematuria*
- *frequency*

---

9   Diagnosis is made by sending three early-morning urine samples for culture (95% detection).

- *urgency*
- *abdominal/loin pain* (due to reflux of infected urine up the ureter)
- *malaise*
- *confusion in the elderly*
- *failure to thrive, poor feeding, incontinence* (paticularly in children).

A UTI may also cause acute *sepsis* with *bacteraemia*.

Investigations

- *Urine dipstick*[10]
- *MSU* for microscopy,[11] *Gram stain* and *culture*
- *Check BM*: diabetes may present with frequency/urgency, and glucosuria (predisposes to infection)
- *Blood tests*: helpful but not always necessary to make diagnosis – *FBC* (elevated WCC), *U&Es* (check electrolytes + renal function), *blood cultures*, *CRP* (elevated).

Further investigations

Further investigations should be undertaken in:

- *children with a UTI*: further investigations include USS and micturating cystogram
- *adult men*: a single proven UTI is likely to be associated with bladder outflow obstruction (consider IVU/flow rate measurements/urodynamics)
- recurrent UTIs.

Treatment

- For a *simple UTI*, the patient may be discharged with a course of *oral antibiotics* (e.g. co-amoxiclav, ciprofloxacin or trimethoprim)
- *Admit for fluid resuscitation* and *intravenous antibiotics* if there is *sepsis*. Admission may also be necessary to treat any underlying cause.

---

10 In the absence of leucocytes and nitrites UTI is unlikely. However, some organisms (e.g. *Pseudomonas*) do not reduce nitrates and consequently give false-negative results. Urine dipstick may be positive in other circumstances, e.g. blood and leucocytes due to appendicitis causing adjacent ureteric inflammation.
11 More than 10^4 leucocytes per ml is significant for a UTI.

Acute pyelonephritis

Definition

Acute pyelonephritis is an infection of the upper urinary tract.

Symptoms

- *Symptoms of UTI*: dysuria, frequency, haematuria
- *Fever/rigors*
- *Flank pain*: usually unilateral and worse on micturition
- *Nausea*
- Occasionally *diarrhoea* and *vomiting*.

However pyelonephritis can be silent, especially in diabetic/immunocompromised patients.

Signs

- *Pyrexia*
- *Tachycardia*
- *Renal angle tenderness.*

Differential diagnosis

- *Renal calculus*
- *Obstructed kidney*
- *Acute glomerulonephritis*
- *Renal infarction*
- *Bleed into a renal tumour/cyst*
- *Renal vein thrombosis*
- *AAA*
- *Cholecystitis*
- *Basal pneumonia.*

Investigations

- *As for a UTI*
- *USS or CT* to confirm diagnosis, exclude obstruction and evaluate any underlying causes.

Treatment

- *Admit*
- *Fluid resuscitation*
- *Analgesia*
- *Antibiotics*: simple pyelonephritis should be treated with a two-week course of antibiotics (e.g. co-amoxiclav or ciprofloxacin). Give i.v. antibiotics if the patient is unwell or cannot tolerate oral antibiotics.

Renal stones and colic

Renal stones

The prevalence of stones is 0.2%. Male:female ratio is 4:1. Incidence is increasing.

Formation of stones

Stones are formed by precipitation of salts in the urine caused by saturation of the inhibitors of crystallisation (citrate, pyrophosphate, and urinary glycoproteins).

Risk factors

Risk factors for stone formation include:

- UTI (especially *Proteus*)
- urinary stasis
- conditions leading to hypercalcaemia (immobility, osteoporosis, hyperparathyroidism, metastatic disease, myeloma, sarcoidosis)
- dehydration
- gout
- primary metabolic disorders, e.g. hypercalciuria
- Crohn's disease
- jejuno-ileal bypass
- laxative abuse
- drugs: loop and thiazide diuretics, antacids, steroids, aspirin, theophyllines.

Types of stone

- *Calcium oxalate*: most common type in the UK (75%). Irregular shape. Associated with Crohn's, chronic diarrhoea and jejuno-ileal bypass
- *Triple phosphate* (calcium magnesium ammonium), or *struvite* (10–20%) These form staghorn calculi. Organisms expressing the urease enzyme (e.g. *Proteus, Klebsiella*) predispose to triple phosphate stone formation
- *Uric acid* (5%): yellow. Can be radiolucent. A quarter of patients with gout develop uric acid stones. Also associated with myeloproliferative disorders
- *Cystine* (1%): very hard stones. Yellow and crystalline. Autosomal recessive inheritance.

Renal colic

Renal colic is pain associated with passage of a stone through the ureter.

Symptoms

- *Severe colicky pain radiating from loin to groin/penis.* Often described as 'worst pain ever'
- *Unable to get comfortable with pain, rolling around*
- *Nausea/vomiting*
- *Urinary frequency.*

Symptoms may be precipitated by dehydration and heavy physical exercise.

Signs

- *Distressed*
- *Renal angle/abdominal tenderness*
- *Palpable kidney* (if obstructed)
- *Fever* suggests co-existing infection
- *Haematuria* (usually microscopic).

Differential diagnosis

- *Biliary colic*
- *Pelviureteric junction (PUJ) obstruction*
- *AAA*
- *Testicular torsion.*

Investigations

- *Urine dipstick*: 90% have microscopic haematuria.[12] In addition look for evidence of infection
- *MSU*: microscopy + culture
- *U&Es*: check electrolytes + renal function
- *FBC*: elevated WCC may indicate co-existing UTI
- *Kidney ureter bladder X-ray (KUB)*: 90% of renal stones are radio-opaque

---

12 Incidence of haematuria declines with time from the onset of pain. *See* Kobayashi T, Nishizawa K, Mitsumori K and Ogura K (2003) Impact of date of onset on the absence of hematuria in patients with acute renal colic. *J Urol* **170**: 1093–6.

- *IVU*: this is the most commonly performed investigation to identify a stone and exclude obstruction
- *Non-contrast CT*:[13] consider if there is a contraindication to IVU (e.g. contrast allergy, patient is asthmatic, or creatinine >200 µmol/l).

Treatment[14]

- *Admit*
- *Fluid resuscitation*
- *Analgesia*: rectal diclofenac (drug of choice unless contraindicated) and pethidine
- *Conservative management may be appropriate* if the stone is <5mm,[15] in the absence of infection or obstruction and where adequate analgesia has been achieved
- *Absolute indications for intervention*:[16] obstruction +/– sepsis, partial obstruction with rising creatinine, or a solitary kidney
- *Relative indications for intervention*: stone >6 mm, ongoing pain, failure of stone to pass spontaneously, staghorn calculus (due to increased risk of sepsis).

Further stone treatment

- *Extracorporeal shock wave lithotripsy (ESWL)*: not possible if the stone is overlying bone. Can cause increase in pain, haematuria, haematoma, and obstruction of the kidney ('Steinstrasse', fragments line up blocking the ureter)
- *Ureteroscopy*, especially for lower third stones which can be fragmented using laser or removed using a Dormia basket
- *Percutaneous nephrolithotomy (PCNL)* for stones in the renal pelvis and proximal ureter
- *Open surgery*: rarely required.

---

13 Non-contrast CT has superseded IVU in many hospitals as the radiological investigation of choice.
14 Whitfield HN (1999) The management of ureteric stones. *Br J Urol Int* **84**: 911–21.
15 >90% of stones less than 5 mm in diameter will pass spontaneously. *See* Segura JW, Preminger GM, Assimos DG *et al.* (1997) Ureteral Stones Clinical Guidelines Panel summary report on the management of ureteral calculi. The American Urological Association. *J Urol* **158**: 1915–21.
16 Ureteric stenting under GA or nephrostomy.

The obstructed kidney

Outflow obstruction leads to reduced glomerular filtration and renal dysfunction.
  Causes include:

- stones (commonest cause)
- malignancy (urinary tract or from surrounding organs)
- congenital obstruction
- stricture
- crossing vessels (lower pole renal artery)
- vesicoureteric reflux
- foreign body
- retroperitoneal fibrosis.

Symptoms

Loin pain. Other symptoms depend on the underlying cause.

Signs

These may include *loin tenderness* and a *palpable kidney. Fever* suggests infection above the level of obstruction.

Investigations

- *Urine dipstick*
- *MSU* for MC&S
- *U&Es*: check electrolytes + renal function
- *FBC*: elevated WCC may indicate co-existing UTI
- Imaging will depend on the likely underlying cause. Consider *USS/IVU* or *CT*.

Treatment

- *Admit*
- *Fluid resuscitation*
- *Analgesia*
- *Urinary catheter* with accurate fluid balance
- *Consider antibiotics*

- *Relieve the obstruction.* If there is evidence of infection then consider drainage by percutaneous nephrostomy. Cover this procedure with antibiotics
- *Further treatment will depend on the underlying cause.*

Pyonephrosis

This is an emergency. The presence of pus in an obstructed kidney can cause rapid irreversible renal damage. Perinephric abscess and sepsis may develop.

Treatment

Resuscitate the patient and administer *i.v. antibiotics.* Arrange *urgent percutaneous nephrostomy.*

Acute scrotum

This is characterised by pain and swelling of the testis and scrotum.

Differential diagnosis

- *Torsion of the testis*
- *Torsion of the hydatid of Morgagni and other appendages of the testis*
- *Epididymo-orchitis*
- *Trauma*
- *Idiopathic scrotal oedema*
- *Inguino-scrotal hernia*
- *Testicular tumour*
- *Hydrocele*
- *Fournier's gangrene.*

Important sources of referred pain to the scrotum

These include:

- *renal colic*
- *leaking AAA*
- *hip pain.*

Torsion of the testis

Incidence

17% of all acute scrotal presentations (accounts for approximately 90% of acute scrotal presentations in adolescents).

Risk factors

Age (peak incidence 14–20 years but can occur in the newborn after a breech delivery), family history, trauma, undescended testis.

Pathogenesis

Rotation of the testis on its cord results in venous congestion and compromise of the arterial supply, with subsequent infarction of the testis. Torsion may be *intravaginal* (rotation of the testis on its cord within the tunica vaginalis), or *extravaginal* (due to an elongated attachment of the tunica vaginalis to the testis). Intravaginal torsion occurs predominantly in adolescents, while extravaginal torsion occurs predominantly in children. There is a higher incidence of torsion in the winter months, and the left side is affected more often than the right.

Symptoms

Sudden onset of *severe pain* in the *scrotum*. Rarely, the pain is felt only in the abdomen (usually the loin of the affected side). Often associated with *nausea* and *vomiting*. There may be a preceding history of trauma.

Signs

- The patient is *distressed*
- Often there is *mild erythema* and *oedema* of the scrotal skin
- The scrotum may have a *bluish tinge* where it overlies the ischaemic testis
- The testis may be *lying horizontally* (the 'bell clapper' testis), and *higher* than its counterpart.

Investigations

No specific investigations are required.[17]

Treatment

- *Admit*
- *NBM*
- *Analgesia*
- *Immediate surgical exploration*[18] of the scrotum is mandatory. A torted testis will remain viable for only 6 h.[19] There must be *no delay* in getting the patient to theatre.

---

17 Doppler ultrasound and radionuclide imaging can be used to assess blood flow to the testis with a high degree of accuracy (90–100%). This may be useful in patients with clinical signs suggestive of epididymitis. However, unless these tests are available on an immediate basis, the patient should be treated on clinical suspicion.

18 Surgery involves detorsion and fixation of the affected testis. Consent the patient for contralateral orchidopexy and possible orchidectomy if the testis is not viable.

19 Testicular salvage rates are over 80% in patients operated within 6 h of the onset of pain. Salvage rates are almost zero after 24 h. *See* Cass AS, Cass BP and Veeraraghavan K (1980) Immediate exploration of the unilateral acute scrotum in young male subjects. *J Urol* **124**: 829–32.

Torsion of the appendages of the testis

Torsion of the hydatid of Morgagni[20] accounts for 90% of cases. This is attached to the front of the upper pole of the testis (it is a vestige of the Müllerian duct).

Risk factors

Pre-adolescents (age 10–12 years is commonest – thought to be due to increased gonadotropins during puberty which increase the size of the hydatid): *see* Figure 10.1 for comparative incidence compared to testicular torsion.

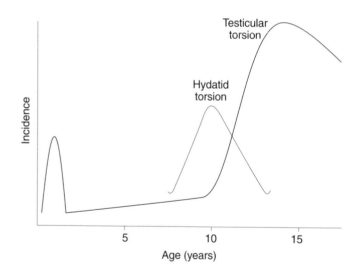

Figure 10.1   Comparative incidence of hydatid and testicular torsion.

Pathogenesis

The hydatid of Morgagni is a pedunculated structure. Rotation of the appendage on its pedicle compromises its blood supply and leads to infarction of the appendage.

---

20 The other appendages are the organ of Giraldes, the vasa aberrantia and the appendix epididymis.

Symptoms

Pain – usually develops insidiously over a period of days.

Signs

- Patient *distressed*
- *Tender scrotum*
- A dark spot may be visible through the scrotal skin in the upper half of the hemiscrotum (the *'blue dot'* sign)
- The *testis* will be *lying normally* in the scrotum
- A *hydrocele* may be present.

Investigations

No specific investigations are required.

Treatment

Surgical exploration is usually necessary to *exclude a torsion*. Once identified, the hydatid is excised. *Conservative treatment* with *scrotal support* and *analgesia* may be considered if the diagnosis is not in doubt.

Acute epididymitis/epididymo-orchitis

Risk factors

Unprotected sexual intercourse, urinary tract pathology[21] (e.g. bladder outflow obstruction).

Pathogenesis

The majority of cases are caused by infection. In younger men (<35 years), the most common infective agents are *Chlamydia trachomatis* and *Neisseria gonorrhoea* introduced to the urinary tract during unprotected sexual intercourse. In older men (>35 years), the most common infective agent is *E. coli*. Some cases are due to viruses (mumps is most common). Approximately one-third of all cases have no identifiable infective cause.

Symptoms

Gradual onset of *pain* and *swelling* in the *scrotum* which develops over several hours or days. Typically, the pain is *constant* and *throbbing* in nature. The majority of patients have associated *fever* and/or *rigors*. Patients may complain of *dysuria* and *urethral discharge*.

Signs

- The majority of patients have a *fever*
- The *epididymis* is *swollen* and extremely *tender* to palpation
- The *testicle* is *tender* in addition to the epididymis in 60% of patients (epididymo-orchitis)
- The *scrotal skin* may be *erythematous* and *oedematous*
- The *testis* will be *lying normally* in the scrotum
- *Late presentation* may result in *abscess formation* which can be difficult to demonstrate clinically because the scrotum and contents are so tender
- *Prostatic enlargement* may be evident on rectal examination.

---

21 Pooling of urine due to urinary tract pathology results in an inability to completely eliminate bacteria from the urinary tract, leading to infection.

Investigations

- *Urine dipstick*: may show nitrites and leucocytes
- *MSU* for microscopy, Gram stain and culture
- *FBC*: elevated WCC
- Consider *urethral swab* for *Chlamydia*
- If an abscess is suspected then an urgent *USS* should be organised.

Treatment

Conservative management with *scrotal support, analgesia* and *antibiotics*. Ofloxacin[22] is the antibiotic of choice in all age groups because it is active against both *Chlamydia* and coliforms. Antibiotics should continue for at least 2 weeks with early follow-up.

NB: If there is any suspicion that the patient has torsion of the testis, or ultrasound has confirmed the presence of an abscess, surgical exploration of the scrotum is mandatory.

---

22 Ofloxacin has better efficacy against *Chlamydia* than other quinolones. *See* Ridgeway GL (1997) Treatment of chlamydial genital infection. *J Antimicrob Chemother* **40**: 311–14.

Idiopathic scrotal oedema

Risk factors

Age: more common in young children and pre-adolescents.

Pathogenesis

Uncertain. Thought to be due to a hypersensitivity reaction that results in angio-oedema of the scrotal skin. However, some believe it may be caused by infection (β-haemolytic *Streptococcus*).

Symptoms

Gradual or sudden onset of *swelling, erythema* and mild *tenderness* of the *scrotum*. Patients are usually well.

Signs

- The patient is *comfortable* with no signs of systemic upset and no tenderness
- It typically involves *one side* but may be bilateral
- Scrotal skin is *erythematous* and *oedematous*
- *Erythema* may extend to involve the *perineum* and *inguinal region*
- The *testes* will be *lying normally* in the scrotum.

Investigations

No specific investigations required but *USS* may help to distinguish from other scrotal pathology.

Treatment

Conservative management with *scrotal support*. The condition will resolve spontaneously in 1 to 2 days. *Antihistamines* may help.

NB: If there is any suspicion that the patient has testicular torsion, surgical exploration of the scrotum is mandatory.

Necrotising fasciitis

This is a potentially deadly soft-tissue infection caused by both aerobic and anaerobic bacteria[23] and associated with fascial necrosis. Muscle and overlying skin are usually spared. Gas gangrene (caused by *Clostridium*) in contrast generally affects muscular tissue and not fascia.

Mortality is approximately 25%.

Risk factors

Diabetes, immunocompromise, i.v. drug abuse.

Causes

- In the *peripheries* it can result from *ulceration*, *trauma*, or *insect bites*
- In the *abdomen* it usually occurs after *'dirty' surgery* or can complicate a *wound infection*. Other causes include a *strangulated hernia*, or after *percutaneous catheterisation*
- In the *perineum*[24] the usual cause is from a *perianal* (particularly ischiorectal) *abscess*.

Symptoms and signs

Diagnosis can be difficult because features are very similar to cellulitis in the first instance. The overlying area is *hot*, *red* and *tender*. *Pain is severe* and is usually out of proportion with physical signs. Following this brief cellulitic period, the area becomes *shiny* and *swollen* before finally becoming *purplish*. There may be *crepitus* of the affected area. Necrosis of the underlying soft tissue leads to what is known as *'dishwater pus'* underneath the skin. After about 5 days the skin becomes *gangrenous* and the patient begins to show signs of *systemic sepsis*.

The disease is usually fatal unless the affected area can be treated early.

---

23 These include Group A *Streptococcus*, *Staphylococcus aureus*, *E. coli*, *Klebsiella*, *Bacteroides*, and occasionally *Vibrio* organisms.
24 Necrotising fasciitis affecting the genitalia is called Fournier's gangrene and can occur after urinary infection or genital trauma.

Investigations

- *Elevated WCC*
- *Elevated CRP*
- *Check U&Es*: electrolytes + renal function
- Occasionally *hypoalbuminaemia, raised glucose, clotting may be deranged*
- *ABGs*: may show metabolic acidosis
- *Blood cultures*
- *MSU* if perineum affected
- *Plain X-ray* of affected area may show gas[25]
- Consider *exploration* or *full-thickness tissue biopsy*
- *CT* or *MRI* may identify soft tissue gas.

Treatment

- *NBM*
- *Fluid resuscitation*
- *Analgesia*
- *Correct coagulopathy prior to surgery*
- *i.v. broad-spectrum antibiotics*: e.g. penicillin, gentamicin and metronidazole. Tailor antibiotics to culture results. Discuss with microbiologists
- *Surgery*: debride all necrotic tissue. Colostomy or amputation may be necessary. The patient should be admitted to ITU following surgery. Surgical re-exploration is usually required at 24 h. Hyperbaric oxygen therapy[26] should be considered if available.

---

25 Gas in the soft tissue on plain X-ray is pathognomonic but is only seen in approximately 50% of patients. *See* Elliott DC, Kufera JA and Myers RA (1996) Necrotizing soft tissue infections. Risk factors for mortality and strategies for management. *Ann Surg* 224: 672–83.

26 Increases tissue oxygen tension in hypoxic areas, thus preventing extension of the disease.

Paraphimosis

Pathogenesis

Paraphimosis occurs when a retracted tight foreskin causes constriction around the subcoronal region of the penis. The prepuce becomes engorged and oedematous, which may lead to gangrene of the glans.

Risk factors

- Iatrogenic (e.g. not replacing the foreskin after urethral catheterisation)
- After sexual intercourse
- Trauma.

Treatment

Manual reduction: pain is minimised by the application of topical anaesthesia.

Compress the glans to reduce the oedema and hook the foreskin back over the glans. The swelling will then subside. An injection of hyaluronidase (150 units) into each side of the prepuce may help reduction.

If manual reduction fails consider:

- *dorsal slit to the foreskin*: this can be performed under penile block (LA). The patient should have a formal circumcision at a later date
- *emergency circumcision* under GA.

As the condition may recur, consider elective circumcision.

Priapism

Priapism is persistent erection of the penis not accompanied by sexual desire.

Pathogenesis

It is either caused by reduced venous outflow from the corpora cavernosa ('low-flow'), or by perineal trauma causing uncontrolled arterial inflow ('high-flow'). 'Low-flow' priapism is more common than 'high-flow'.

Causes

- *Sickle-cell disease*[27]
- *Gout*
- *Thrombophilia* and other haematological disorders
- *Drugs*: anticoagulants, anti-hypertensives, centrally acting drugs
- *Hormonal treatment.*

Treatment

Low-flow priapism

- *Oxygen*
- *Fluid resuscitation*
- *Analgesia* (i.v. opioids or penile local anaesthetic block)
- *Ice and elevation*
- Oral or subcutaneous *terbutaline* may be helpful
- Consider injection of an α-*adrenergic agonist* into the corpora cavernosa (e.g. phenylephrine). Methylene blue injection is an alternative (inhibits cyclic GMP)
- *Surgery* is indicated if the above treatments fail. This involves construction of a cavernosal-spongiosum anastomosis.

High-flow priapism

This usually requires *angiography* and *embolisation* of the responsible vessels.

---

27 Up to 40% of adults with sickle-cell disease will have an episode of priapism in their lifetime.

Chapter 11

Important paediatric surgical emergencies

Intussusception

Intussusception occurs when part of the bowel invaginates into an adjacent lower segment (77% are ileocolic). 90% are associated with lymphoid hyperplasia of Peyer's patches in the terminal ileum.

Incidence

4:1000 (male predominance of 2:1).

Age range

Usually occurs between 2 and 24 months.

Symptoms and signs

- *Paroxysmal pain* associated with drawing up of the legs
- *Vomiting*
- *Distended abdomen*
- *Blood-stained mucus rectally* ('redcurrant jelly stool'). This is a late and often absent feature
- *Palpable sausage-shaped mass* in the abdomen.

Investigations

- *Plain AXR*: mass, absent gas pattern in RIF
- *Abdominal USS* may be helpful.[1]

Treatment

- *Resuscitation*
- *Hydrostatic* or *pneumatic radiological reduction*[2]
- *Surgery* is necessary in the event of perforation, peritonitis or following failed radiological reduction.

---

1 Verschelda P, Filiatrault D and Garel L (1992) Intussusception in children: reliability of ultrasound in diagnosis – a prospective study. *Radiology* **184**: 741–4.
2 British Society of Paediatric Radiology (1999) Guidelines for intussusception reduction. *See* www.bspr.org.uk/intuss.htm (accessed 7 November 2005).

Hernias

In male infants indirect inguinal hernias (and hydroceles) result from a patent processus vaginalis and are slightly more common on the right side. Direct hernias are rare. An inguinal hernia is the commonest cause of intestinal obstruction in neonates.

Incidence

4% of male infants.

Age range

Most common in the first 3 months of life. Uncommon after the age of 3 years.

Complications

There is a high risk of incarceration and strangulation in the first year of life.

Treatment of an incarcerated hernia

- Attempt *manual reduction*. If this is successful then observe the patient in hospital
- If reduction is unsuccessful, *surgical repair* is indicated
- If there is evidence of strangulation, *surgery* is mandatory following resuscitation.

Pyloric stenosis

This is an inherited condition that results in hypertrophy of the circular muscles of the pylorus.

Incidence

4:1000. M>F. Most common in first-born child.

Age range

In the first 4–6 weeks of life.

Symptoms and signs

- *Non-bilious projectile vomiting*
- *Failure to thrive despite hunger*
- *Visible peristalsis*
- *Palpable 'walnut' mass* deep to the right rectus in the transpyloric plane.

Investigations

- *Check U&Es*: hyponatraemia, hypokalaemia, hypochloridaemia
- *Capillary blood gases*: metabolic alkalosis
- *Abdominal USS* will confirm the diagnosis.

Treatment

- *Fluid resuscitation* with correction of electrolytes/alkalosis
- *Pyloromyotomy* when the child is stable.

Necrotising enterocolitis

This is thought to be due to ischaemia of the large bowel wall with translocation of luminal bacteria resulting in systemic sepsis. Mortality is high.

Age range

Newborn babies.

Symptoms and signs

- *Fever*
- *Bilious vomiting*
- *Bloody diarrhoea*
- *Abdominal distension*
- *Generalised peritonitis* may occur following *perforation*.

Investigations

- *FBC*: leucocytosis
- *AXR* may show a thickened dilated bowel wall containing intramural gas.

Treatment

- *Fluid resuscitation*
- *Broad-spectrum antibiotics*
- *Surgical resection* of necrotic bowel may be needed.

These patients should be managed in the paediatric ICU.

Malrotation of the gut

Malrotation is a congenital problem usually affecting the midgut. It can cause duodenal obstruction (secondary to Ladd's bands) in the neonate or recurrent volvulus in older children.

Pre-operative considerations

- A child should not be starved pre-operatively for any longer than the normal interval between feeds or for 4 h in older children
- All drugs and fluids should be prescribed according to weight (not age)
- Aim for a urine output of at least 1 ml/kg/h
- Normal fluid requirements are:
  - child up to 10 kg, 100 ml/kg/day
  - child 10–20 kg, 1 l + 50 ml/kg/day
  - child >20 kg, 1.5 l + 25 ml/kg/day
- In shock, 20 ml/kg bolus of saline should be used as a fluid challenge.

Appendix 1

Common reference intervals

Haematology

Table A1.1

Parameter	Reference range	Units
Haemoglobin (Hb)	12.5–18.0 (male)	g/dl
	11.5–16.0 (female)	g/dl
Haematocrit (Hct)	37.0–54.0 (male)	%
	33.0–47.0 (female)	%
Mean cell volume (MCV)	80.0–100.0	fl
Platelets (PLTS)	150–400	$\times 10^9$/l
White blood cell count (WBC)	3.5–11.0	$\times 10^9$/l
Neutrophils (NEUT)	2.0–7.5	$\times 10^9$/l
Lymphocytes (LYMPH)	1.0–3.5	$\times 10^9$/l
Eosinophils (EOSIN)	0.0–0.4	$\times 10^9$/l
Erythrocyte sedimentation rate (ESR)	<10 (male)	mm in 1 h
	<20 (female)	mm in 1 h
Prothrombin time (PT)	10.6–14.9	s
Activated partial thromboplastin time (APTT)	23.0–35.0	s
Thrombin time (TT)	10.5–15.5	s
D-Dimer	<0.25	µg/ml
Fibrinogen	1.5–3.8	g/l

Biochemistry

Table A1.2

Parameter	Reference range	Units
Sodium	135–145	mmol/l
Potassium	3.5–5.0	mmol/l
Urea	2.5–7.0	mmol/l
Creatinine	50–130	μmol/l
Magnesium	0.75–1.00	mmol/l
Total bilirubin (bili)	2–17	μmol/l
Alanine aminotransferase (ALT)	<35	U/l
Aspartate transaminase (AST)	<45	U/l
Alkaline phosphatase (ALP)	35–125	U/l
Albumin	36–52	g/l
Calcium	2.2–2.6	mmol/l
Phosphate	0.7–1.4	mmol/l
Amylase	<200	U/l
Glucose (random)	<11.1	mmol/l
Glucose (fasting)	3.5–5.5	mmol/l

Arterial blood gases

Table A1.3

Parameter	Reference range	Units
pH[1]	7.35–7.45	
PO$_2$	11.9–13.2	kPa
PCO$_2$	4.8–6.3	kPa
Base excess	±2	mmol/l

Table A1.4 Simplified changes to arterial blood gas parameters in different acid–base disturbances

Acid–base problem	pH	PaCO$_2$	Standard bicarbonate
Respiratory acidosis	Low	High	Normal or high
Respiratory alkalosis	High	Low	Normal or high
Metabolic acidosis	Low	Normal or low	Low
Metabolic alkalosis	High	Normal	High

---

1 Arterial blood pH is closely regulated around the pH 7.4 mark. Hydrogen ions produced by metabolising cells are buffered by proteins, but also by haemoglobin. Furthermore, plasma bicarbonate can mop up hydrogen ions producing CO$_2$, which is then exhaled.

Appendix 2

In-hospital resuscitation and Advanced life support

In-hospital resuscitation

For any patient who collapses whilst in hospital follow the algorithm as shown in Figure A2.1.

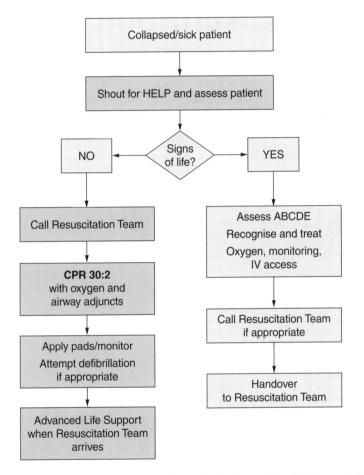

Figure A2.1 Algorithm for in-hospital resuscitation. Reproduced with permission from the UK Resuscitation Council.

Advanced life support (ALS)

The protocol for the management of cardiac arrest in adults is shown in Figure A2.2.

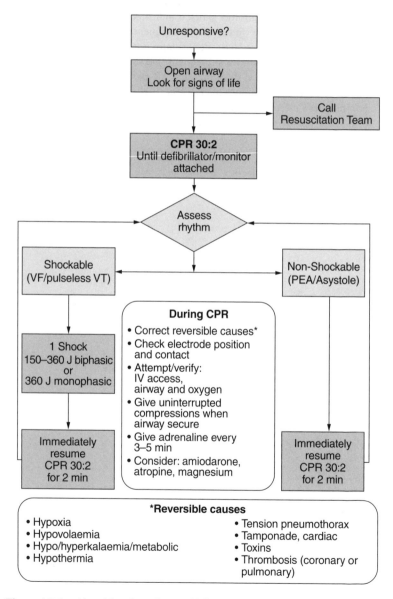

Figure A2.2   Algorithm for advanced life support in adults. Reproduced with permission from the UK Resuscitation Council.

Important points regarding the ALS algorithm[1]

- Early defibrillation during a cardiac arrest is the most important manoeuvre.
- Treat ventricular fibrillation (VF)/pulseless ventricular tachycardia (VT) with a single shock followed by resumption of CPR for 2 minutes. After 2 minutes of CPR give another shock if indicated from the rhythm.
- Use 360 J for both the initial and subsequent shocks if a *monophasic* defibrillator is used. If a *biphasic* defibrillator is used then 150–200 J for the first shock and 150–360 J for subsequent shocks.
- Give 1 mg adrenaline i.v. if VF/pulseless VT persists after a second shock and repeat every 3–5 minutes if VF/VT persists.
- For pulseless electrical activity/asystole give 1 mg adrenaline i.v. once intravenous access is established and repeat every 3–5 minutes until rhythm change.
- There is some evidence that induction of hypothermia during cardiac arrest may improve survival.

---

1   There are important changes in the new ALS guidelines published December 2005 by the UK Resuscitation Council. See www.resus.org.uk/pages/als.pdf

Index

Page numbers in *italic* refer to figures or tables.